PAEDIATRIC INTENSIVE CARE

Paediatric Intensive Care

A Manual for Resident Medical Officers and Senior Nurses

KEITH D. ROBERTS
Ch.M. (Birm.) F.R.C.S. (Eng.)
Consultant Cardio-thoracic Surgeon,
Children's Hospital, United Birmingham Hospitals
Honorary Consultant Thoracic Surgeon,
Birmingham Regional Hospital Board
Clinical Lecturer in Surgery,
University of Birmingham

JENNIFER M. EDWARDS
M.B., B.S (Adel.) F.F.A., R.A.C.S.(Melb.)
Consultant Anaesthetist,
Children's Hospital, United Birmingham Hospitals
Clinical Lecturer in Anaesthetics
University of Birmingham

BLACKWELL SCIENTIFIC PUBLICATIONS
OXFORD AND EDINBURGH

© 1971 by Blackwell Scientific Publications
5 Alfred Street, Oxford, England and
9 Forrest Road, Edinburgh, Scotland

All rights reserved. No part of this publication
may be reproduced, stored in a retrieval system,
or transmitted, in any form or by any means,
electronic, mechanical, photocopying, recording
or otherwise without the prior permission of
the copyright owner.

ISBN 0 632 08020 5

First published 1971

Distributed in the U.S.A. by
F. A. Davis Company, 1915 Arch Street,
Philadelphia, Pennsylvania

Printed and bound in Great Britain by
C. Tinling & Co., London and Prescot

RJ
245
.R6

Contents

Introduction
A. L. d'Abreu, C.B.E., Ch.M., (Birm.) F.R.C.S. (Eng.)
F.R.C.P. (Lond.) *Barling Professor of Surgery, University of Birmingham*

1	The Concept of Intensive Patient Care	1
2	Design Features	5
3	Infection, Cross-Infection and Sterilisation	15
4	Fluid, Electrolyte and Metabolic Balance	21
5	Acid/Base Balance and Blood Gas Studies	47
6	Respiratory Physiology	60
7	Cardiovascular Physiology	73
8	Patient Monitoring	91

G. Hall Davies, M.B., Ch.B., (Birm.) F.F.A.R.C.S. (Eng.), *Consultant Anaesthetist, The Children's Hospital, Birmingham, Clinical Lecturer in Anaesthetics, University of Birmingham.*

9	Ventilators	105
10	Radiological Investigations	125

F G. O. Burrows, F.R.S.C. (Eng.), D.M.R.D. (Eng.), F.F.R. *Consultant Radiologist, The Children's Hospital, Birmingham. Clinical Lecturer in Radiology, University of Birmingham.*

11 The Nurse in the I.T.U.	134
Miss S. Barton, S.R.N., R.S.C.N., *Sister-in-Charge, I.T.U., The Children's Hospital, Birmingham.*	
12 Care of Respiratory Problems	148
13 Post-operative Thoracic Surgical Care	169
14 Cardiovascular Management	180
15 Acute Renal Failure	199
R. H. R. White, M.A. (Cantab), M.D. (Birm.), M.R.C.P. (Lond.), D.C.H. (Eng.), *Consultant Paediatrician, The Children's Hospital, Birmingham. Clinical Lecturer in Paediatrics, University of Birmingham.*	
16 Special Problems of Neonates	218
17 Convulsive States and the Unconscious Patient	232
18 Emergency Resuscitation	245
Appendix	
Doses of drugs commonly used in the I.T.U.	255
Index	261

Preface

In a time of increasing interest in 'intensive patient care' and 'progressive patient care' we feel that the appearance of yet another book on the subject perhaps requires an explanation, but certainly not an apology!

The present work is based in part on lectures given during the 'Intensive Therapy Course' of the United Birmingham Hospitals. It has become increasingly apparent that, in the treatment of patients requiring specialised care, there is the need for cooperation and communication between medical and nursing staff much closer than in the ordinary ward environment, and it is vital that everyone 'speaks the same language'. We believe that the intensive therapy unit creates more physical and psychological demands on the nurse than in any other hospital area, and, if stress is to be minimised, the nurse must receive proper support from the medical staff.

We regard the I.T.U. nurse as one combining the attributes of a 'medical' nurse, a 'surgical' nurse, and a 'theatre' nurse. She must be capable of reaching decisions rapidly and basing her actions on experience and logical reasoning. In her own field she must be able to interpret and act, in a highly intelligent and sophisticated way, on the complex data with which she is presented. On occasion we have found junior medical staff obtaining advice from a senior I.T.U. sister about management of a particular problem, and indeed, there is nothing invidious in that. It seems to us that there is a need to make clear both to resident doctors and senior nurses the basic principles underlying the care of the critically ill child, and we trust that we have not been too ambitious in our attempt to provide a practical manual for both. While the contents may emphasise the care of the cardiorespiratory systems, these after all have fundamental importance in the preservation of life. We have deliberately adopted a somewhat pragmatic approach, and references have been omitted. The methods and techniques described are those with which the authors are personally familiar, and which are in current use in their own unit. It is obviously impossible to consider the detailed management of particular conditions, and indeed, that is not our purpose. We have endeavoured to provide basic information on which logical management of a particular problem can be based.

We are indebted to many past teachers, present colleagues and nursing staff for ideas which have been included, and it would be impossible to thank these individually. We do, however, wish to express our appreciation to Miss Rozanne Craig, for typing the manuscript, a task over which she has laboured with the greatest energy and good humour.

Lastly, we would stress that we have learnt and continue to learn by observation of the patient, and it is to the care of the sick child that this book is dedicated.

K.D.R.
J.M.E.

Introduction

It is said, probably correctly, that all neonates after surgery require Intensive Care; certainly all neonates and older children undergoing thoracic and cardiac surgery need such provision.

Mr. Keith Roberts, before he became a consultant, worked with me as a registrar and senior registrar in thoracic surgery. To an operative skill of the highest quality, he added great expertise in the immediate pre-operative and post-operative care of his and my patients. Having acquired a wide experience both of adult and paediatric thoracic and cardio-vascular surgery, he eventually decided to concentrate on the paediatric side of this work. He has an extensive experience of the difficult problems in this field, in which he is now a recognised authority.

When questions are asked as to who should control intensive care units, answers vary; the ideal solution is to find anaesthetists and surgeons who will share this heavy burden and they in turn will seek assistance from other colleagues such as physicians, radiologists and clinical biochemists in addition to high quality nursing personnel. The Birmingham Children's Hospital has been fortunate to have Mr. Roberts and Dr. Jennifer Edwards collaborating with their colleagues in the compilation of this fine manual. Dr. G. Hall Davies, Dr. F. G. O. Burrows, Miss Barton and Dr. R. H. R. White have written chapters on patient monitoring, radiological investigations, nursing care, data recording and renal failure. Such co-operation underlines the need to treat those rapid fluctuations in the physiopathological behaviour of patients who have undergone surgical operations on the thorax, and which provide such dangerous changes of homeostasis that more than one or two experts may be needed at any time of the day or night to apply their specialised knowledge, advice and help. I have much enjoyed reading the manuscript which is written and illustrated lucidly; when detail is required, it is carefully stated. I am confident that this manual will be of great value to those concerned with the care of seriously ill neonates and children.

A. L. d'Abreu
Barling Professor of Surgery,
University of Birmingham.

Grant me strength, time and opportunity always to correct what I have acquired, always to extend its domain; for knowledge is immense and the spirit of man can extend infinitely to enrich itself daily with new requirements. Today he can discover his errors of yesterday and tomorrow he may obtain a new light on what he thinks himself sure of today.

Maimonides

CHAPTER

1

The Concept of Intensive Patient Care

It is usually considered that the idea of concentrating ill patients in a small area with a large number of nurses to care for them is relatively modern. However, Florence Nightingale in 1863 wrote: 'It is not uncommon, in small country hospitals, to have a recess or small room leading from the operating theatre, in which patients remain until they have recovered, or at least recovered from the immediate effects of the operation.' ('Notes on Hospitals'). This was the forerunner of the post-operative recovery room, which, together with experience of special surveillance units in the Second World War, and experience of treating respiratory paralysis during the poliomyelitis epidemic in Scandinavia in 1952–53, led to the practice of grouping critically ill patients together *irrespective of the nature of their disease or trauma*. In the case of poliomyelitis, it was found that these patients, who were seriously ill and requiring the use of ventilators and monitoring equipment, were better looked after by persons who understood the use of the apparatus, and by having such patients together it was possible to reduce the mortality.

The patient in need of intensive care requires the ordinary recordings of temperature, pulse and respiratory rate, made more frequently than in the ordinary ward environment, together with more technical observations such as acid/base determinations carried out as often as necessary. Based on observation of the patient and examination of the data collected, special mechanical or electronic support of the patient's vital functions may be necessary until the disease process is arrested or improved. Patients may thus require artificial pulmonary ventilation, peritoneal or haemodialysis, cardiac pacing, or correction of a severe metabolic upset. Moreover, they do not often suffer derangement of *one* body system; for example, impaired cardiac output may bring pulmonary, renal and metabolic complications.

It must be stressed that an intensive therapy unit is *not* to be used to relieve the load of nursing an ill patient on the ordinary ward unless the additional facilities are necessary.

There is no virtue and every disadvantage in having a multiplicity of intensive care areas within one hospital, such as a 'medical' and a 'surgical' intensive therapy unit. In so far as *management* is concerned there is little difference in the care of a patient who is ventilating his lungs inadequately after cerebral trauma compared with one who has sustained cerebral anoxia due to cardiac arrest, while the therapeutic plan for management of tetanus is not very different from that required for status epilepticus. A multiplicity of units defeats the intention to conserve medical and nursing resources.

The criterion for admission to an intensive therapy unit *must* be the need for the patient to have the advantage of the special skills available. For this reason we accept the need to nurse the infectious patient within the unit, and such a case should not be discharged to an isolation block if still requiring special care, but obviously special precautions will be necessary to reduce the risk of cross infection.

Although conventionally an intensive therapy unit is described in terms of the number of beds, related to the total number of hospital beds, it is important to realise that it should really be considered in terms of *space*. Each patient requires a greater floor space than is often found in the ordinary ward as he may be surrounded by items of bulky equipment. In addition, the whole unit requires an area, equal to the patient area, devoted to the storage of disposable equipment, dressing packs, ventilators, electronic monitors, etc.

In a paediatric hospital of 250 beds a reasonable number to be devoted to intensive care would be 10, half of these being for infants. It is essential that administration within the unit should be by one member of the consultant staff, with a deputy. It really does not matter whether the director is a physician, surgeon or anaesthetist, provided he is able to devote sufficient time to the organisation of the unit, although, since many of the problems are respiratory there is much to be said for control by an anaesthetist. The fact that there is a clinical director of the unit *should not* mean that patients admitted to the unit are removed from the clinical care of the consultant under whom they were originally treated. We feel that it is important that the administrative director of the unit does not usurp the responsibilities of the clinician in charge of any particular patient, and that there is really no place for the specialist 'intensivist' who takes over the care of a patient completely. In our view an 'intensivist' cannot have the knowledge in depth of all problems likely to arise, and it is better for the director of the unit to act as a coordinator, if necessary, of the various disciplines that may be concerned in the care of an individual patient. It is equally important that a patient is not treated by a committee! During any twenty four hours period decisions may have to be taken for immediate changes in management which cannot be referred back for approval, and this principle must be accepted by the hospital staff. The decision to admit a patient to, or discharge from, the unit must rest with the clinical director, who must relate such a request to the work load within the intensive care ward. Even if there is a vacant space it may not be possible to increase the load on the nursing staff who may be working to capacity; to admit another patient in such circumstances means not only that the new arrival cannot receive all the care necessary, but also that the patients already present would suffer from lack of sufficient care. If the unit is already full, a request for a further admission may have to be refused, or a decision made to discharge a patient back to the general ward to make room for the new arrival. Such decisions are never easy and should not be expected of a registrar or the sister in charge of the unit.

Since the management of the patient depends on the collection of data, which may have to be repeated frequently, it is desirable that the unit contains a laboratory where estimations of blood gases, for example, can be done without delay and almost at the bed side.

As is the case in any unit where advanced treatment is carried out, nurses in an intensive therapy unit are required to undertake tasks that previously have been considered the responsibility of the medical staff, and indeed, the criticism is sometimes made that the I.T.U. nurse is becoming a technician and replaces the need for a doctor. However, provided a particular task is one which the nurse has been taught and is competent to do, and the head of nursing services and employing authority are aware of this position, properly prepared nurses, understanding their personal responsibilities, can well undertake this advanced clinical role. We stress our belief that I.T.U.s require highly skilled, intelligent nurses who are capable of rapid reaction to changing situations based on experience and reasoning from observed data. Success in patient care will not be achieved if the nurse lacks initiative and decisiveness. There is perhaps no greater nursing challenge than the bedside care of the desperately ill patient in an I.T.U.

With regard to student nurses we feel that it is useful as part of a student's education for her to spend a portion of her training in the I.T.U. where, however, she would be *extra* to the nursing team and not considered as part of the nursing establishment. A student nurse should be allowed to carry out certain procedures under supervision, and not be a mere observer. It is useful for a clinical teacher to be part of the nursing team provided it is recognised that she does not form part of the establishment with service commitments.

Junior medical staff should not be asked to accept responsibility in an I.T.U. until they have been introduced to the work under supervision and their competence assessed. It is most desirable that registrars should work in rotation in an I.T.U., and such experience applies equally to anaesthetic, medical and surgical residents. Patients in an I.T.U. may require continuous or immediately available medical attention and it has been suggested that this requires two additional senior house officers. If this is not possible, a workable compromise is a rota system by which one suitably experienced doctor is made available at all times of a twenty four hour period to give absolute priority to the demands of the unit. The junior medical staffing of an I.T.U. will obviously depend on the local situation, but however medical cover is achieved it is most important to have a regular daily round attended by medical and nursing staff and at which the broad policy concerning each patient over the next twenty four hours can be discussed.

FURTHER READING

Intensive Care. B.M.A. Planning Unit Report No. 1. November, 1967.
Intensive Therapy Units. Royal College of Nursing Intensive Therapy Nursing Group 1969.

CHAPTER 2

Design Features

An intensive therapy unit may be defined as a hospital area providing a *facility* giving more space, staff and equipment for the care of a patient than is possible in the ordinary ward environment, and a *service* providing continuous observation of vital functions, and support of those functions more efficiently than is possible in the general ward.

The I.T.U. should *not* form part of the operating theatre suite although it may conveniently be situated adjacent to this.

Certain fundamental principles must be defined before considering the most efficient design of an I.T.U.

Number of beds
It has been estimated that 1 per cent of patients admitted to a hospital will require intensive therapy at some time. Probably a proportion of four beds in the I.T.U. per 100 beds in the hospital as a whole, is workable, and it must be remembered that bed occupancy in an I.T.U. may well be lower than that in a general ward because of fluctuations in work load. An I.T.U. of less than 5 beds is uneconomic and one of more than 15 beds is unwieldy and unrealistic in terms of availability of skilled nursing and supporting staff. Probably a good average number of beds is 10. If the hospital is large enough to require more than 15 I.T.U. beds it is probably better to have two I.T.U. areas side by side with a common administration so that interchange between the two units can be arranged without difficulty.

Staffing

An I.T.U. is staffed by medical and nursing personnel, together with nursing aides and domestic staff. Ultimate clinical responsibility is vested in the consultant medical staff, but continuity of management of the patient lies in the hands of trained nursing staff who *may* be more competent to deal with a particular situation than a junior doctor who may be inexperienced, or who may only have worked in the unit for a short time. The nursing situation is outlined in Chapter 11, but it must be emphasised that the presence of an I.T.U. in a hospital is *not* a means of remedying an overall nurse shortage, nor is it a hospital area which is economical to run in terms of trained nursing staff.

Type of patient

All patients requiring intensive therapy should be brought together within one area of the hospital, and the use of the unit should be restricted to those patients who require continuous nursing. Thus patients who have had multiple injuries or major surgery, or who require maintenance of an adequate airway, or whose cardiovascular integrity requires maintenance, or who require treatment of toxaemia of metabolic or infective origin, may all be considered as suitable cases *because they are severely ill*. Infection should *not* be a bar to admission to an I.T.U., and indeed may be the reason for admission, but special provision must be made for such patients.

Location of the Unit

Ideally this should be on the same floor as the operating theatre, which has advantages both for ready access to the unit of patients returning from the operating theatre (and for patients to return to the operating theatre if further emergency procedures are necessary), and also for the provision of essential services.

Work pattern of the Unit

In most instances specialization depends on the work load of the hospital concerned, and to some extent the interest and work of the consultant or consultants who started a particular unit. Owing to the fluctuations in demand for the service of an I.T.U. it is desirable that it should have a link with a special field such as cardiovascular surgery. This means that if bed occupancy of the I.T.U. is low at any particular time, the beds can be filled by an increase of planned procedures, thus avoiding a period of frustration amongst the nursing staff due to inactivity. For example, a purely 'respiratory unit' in a children's hospital will have a marked seasonal variation in the demands made on it so that at times it will be almost unoccupied. Whatever the particular interest of the consultants in charge of the unit may be (e.g. cardiology, anaesthetics etc.), provision must be made for the care of *all* types of illness, so that the unit must be able to cope with peritoneal dialysis as well as post-operative cardiothoracic surgery, and with status epilepticus as well as head injuries. Admission to the unit by the consultant in charge, or his deputy, is based solely on the patient's need, and the consultant in administrative charge should have the ultimate decision concerning admissions and discharges. The clinical responsibility of care of an individual patient rests with the consultant under whose care the patient was admitted to hospital; the organisation of the *service* (e.g. provision of measures for emergency resuscitation, or artificial ventilation) does not clash with other aspects of patient care, and minute-to-minute details of patient management must be left to the I.T.U. staff.

General Layout of the Patient Area

Much controversy exists concerning the arrangement of beds within the I.T.U. area, and there are advocates of all beds being contained within single cubicles, while in contradistinction some clinicians prefer a completely open ward. The advantage of cubicles is *said* to be the reduction of cross infection hazards, but in practice there must always be *some* breakdown of 'barrier nursing' even when patients are in individual cubicles. A disadvantage of complete segregation of patients is that when they are beginning to recover from the condition necessitating their admission to the I.T.U., they feel emotionally 'cut off' and this is particularly so in young children. Perhaps the best solution is a compromise, in which the patient area is divided up. For example, in an I.T.U. of ten beds, there could be two cubicles each for one or two patients with a multi-bed area for six patients. It is imperative that the nurse at a central nursing station should be able to observe *all* the patients, so that any partitions must be glazed with transparent material in the upper half. The exact location of each bed will vary according to the wishes of individual units, but each patient area *must* contain sufficient space to allow use of bulky equipment, space for manoeuvre and adequate space for the numerous members of the team to work. Designs have been produced for the patient area varying from a long oblong, or a square, to a circular unit with beds radiating from a central nursing station.

The central nursing station is essentially a place where there is a desk, x-ray viewing boxes, storage for radiographs and notes and several seats. There is a widespread belief that a central nursing station should have a vast multichannel panel which records data obtained from each patient, and which can be watched by a nurse seated at the console. *Nothing is further from correct I.T.U. practice.* While 'repeater' monitors at the central nursing station may have some uses, they cannot and should not replace observation of the patient and his individual monitoring apparatus, ventilator etc. by the trained nurse *at the bed side*.

The position of the patient at each patient station may be either head to wall or feet to wall according to convenience. Thus it may be easier to have a respiratory problem treated by artificial ventilation nursed feet-to-wall. It is extremely important to position equipment in the most economical way with regard to space, so that it is useful to have shelving or rails on the walls where equipment can be placed. It is desirable to avoid the use of 'drip stands' for infusions by hanging intravenous infusion bottles from an overhead bar.

If, as suggested, the patient area is subdivided, one subdivision is usefully employed as an initial treatment room where the intensive therapy régime can be begun. After some improvement in the patient's condition has occurred he can be transferred to the multi-bed area. Similarly, the infected case can be partially segregated and a strict barrier nursing procedure applied.

In a children's hospital the I.T.U. should be capable of managing neonates, infants, toddlers and older children. Flexibility is thus mandatory. While many infants can be nursed in incubators, this having the theoretical advantage that they are living in their own clean (or dirty!) environment, this is by no means always necessary or even convenient; for example it is difficult to treat an infant attached to a ventilator if he is lying in an incubator, and it may be preferable to have him in an open bassinette with some form of overhead heating (e.g. infra-red lamps) to prevent loss of body heat.

Equipment which is needed for immediate use must be stored in the

Design Features

patient area so that it is readily to hand; for example, drugs must be accessible. Much of the routinely used materials such as intravenous infusion sets, syringes and needles, suction catheters etc. are disposable, while the remainder of the equipment, e.g. intravenous 'cut-down' instruments, tracheostomy packs, will be provided from the central sterile supply department. Although enough equipment should be available in the patient area for hour-by-hour use, it is obvious that a larger stock must be held as a reserve. It is thus essential to have a storage room where additional C.S.S.D. and disposable supplies can be kept, together with such items as spare linen, ventilators, spare incubators, oxygen tents etc. *It is important to have a storage area equal in size to the patient area.*

Lighting is extremely important so that adequate observation of the patient is possible at all times. Each bed area should be capable of illumination from the ceiling to a maximum of 30 lumens per square foot (300 lux) at bed level. Multi-strip fluorescent lighting is the most convenient, and glare to the patient must be minimized by careful siting of the light fittings; individual dimming devices should be available so that lighting can be adjusted to a low intensity if required. If a higher intensity of light is required for some procedure to be carried out, a powerful portable light source should be used. Low level lighting is also necessary to allow inspection of drainage bottles etc.

In spite of the fact that an I.T.U. is supplied largely with disposable and C.S.S.D. items, it is useful to have a small portable electrically heated pressure steam steriliser 175 mm diameter x 300 mm length for emergency use. The most convenient location for this will depend on the individual unit's general layout.

ANCILLARY ROOMS

While the patient area and the storage room mentioned above are the most important areas in the unit, certain other rooms are almost as essential. These include a staff lounge/changing room, a cleaner's room, a dirty utility sluice, a staff lavatory, a relatives' room, a laboratory, and possibly a doctor's room.

Staff lounge/changing room
This room can serve a variety of functions. In addition to containing lockers and a supply of I.T.U. uniform dresses, there should be

facilities for the preparation of light snacks and beverages. *Comfortable* chairs are essential, and it must be possible for a nurse working under stress with a difficult case to be relieved for a short period of time so that she can have a rest and some refreshment. A further use of this room is for discussion of problems of administration and technical procedures, which can take place between medical and nursing staff at times when the unit load is less heavy.

Cleaner's room
This room is most necessary, and must be equipped with hot and cold water, and necessary cleaning materials with space for such items as mechanical aids to cleaning. Repeated cleaning of the unit is important as a means of limiting cross-infection risks, but must be carried out in a non-dust-raising manner.

Dirty utility/sluice room
Dirty and used goods can be stored here pending cleaning, or disposal, or transfer to the C.S.S.D. In addition, provision must be made for cleaning of such items as chest drainage bottles and tubing, cleaning and sterilization of bed pans and urine bottles, or facilities for disposal of these if they are disposable. There must be facilities for urine testing and storage of specimens of urine, faeces etc. before removal to the appropriate laboratory.

Relatives' room
This room is preferably sited adjacent to the I.T.U. area itself, and should be suitably furnished. It is also used for interviewing relatives. Visitors to the unit itself will don gowns in the lobby before actually entering the unit.

Laboratory
A small laboratory is essential for certain procedures to be carried out on the spot, and should be equipped with a laboratory sink and bench, storage cupboards, electrical sockets etc. It is particularly useful for blood gas and acid/base balance determination to be done in the unit itself. More routine haemotological and biochemical investigations should be done in the hospital's central laboratories.

Doctor's room
This room is useful for the doctor on duty in the unit to employ as an

Design Features

office if required. It is controversial as to whether it should be used as a bedroom at night. With properly trained nursing staff if a doctor is required at night he should be up and working in the unit not sleeping there. The only reason for having a doctor sleeping in the unit should be if the hospital residences are situated at a considerable distance away from the I.T.U.

Other rooms which can be provided if space is allowed, but which are not essential, include one for the sister-in-charge of the unit, which can be used for interviewing staff and preparing reports, and a small workshop for minor servicing of ventilators and electronic equipment.

PROVISION AND SITING OF ENGINEERING SERVICES

The proper management of patients in an I.T.U. is dependent to a great extent on the efficient and uninterrupted use of machines and equipment upon which the life of the patient may depend. Several pieces of apparatus may be in use on an individual patient at the same time, and in an emergency further items may be required. It is thus essential to have sufficient service fixtures at each bed station to cover all eventualities.

Piped supplies

Piped oxygen with two outlets is required at each bed station, with suitable flow meters, each outlet being capable of delivery of 20 litres/minute at a pressure of 60 pounds p.s.i. The oxygen should preferably come from the hospital's main reservoir tank, otherwise two banks of cylinders are necessary with a warning system and automatic change-over control.

Compressed air should be available with one outlet and flow meter for each bed. If the air is supplied by a compressor the air must be filtered, dried and oil free.

Piped vacuum is essential as a means of providing suction for tracheo-bronchial aspiration, and for providing assistance to drainage bottles (for example, pleural drains). Two outlets with manometers are necessary at each bed, and air extraction should be 40 litres/minute when the vacuum in the pipeline is 500 mm Hg below standard barometric pressure of 760 mm Hg. It is important to interpose two empty bottles as a trap between the patient and the vacuum

line to avoid drawing water, secretions etc. over into the vacuum line
and pump (see Fig. 2.1).

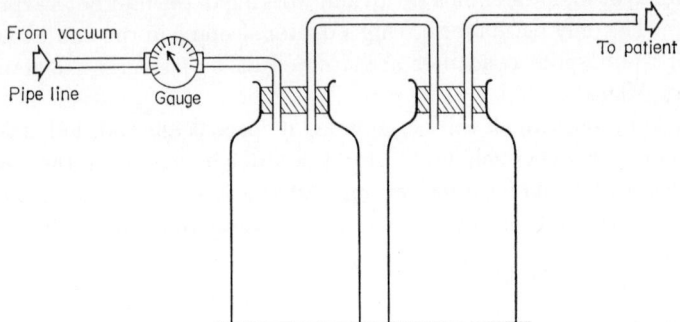

FIG. 2.1   Arrangement of vacuum line.

Power

Town gas should be provided only in the laboratory as it constitutes
a fire hazard. The beverage bay in the staff lounge should have suitable electrical appliances. Socket outlets for electronic equipment
must also be provided in the laboratory. At each bed station eight
single socket outlets should be provided, preferably 13 amp. switched
and shuttered. It is most important that all sockets should be
standardised so that any item of equipment can be used at any
socket. A special 13 amp. plug is available which accommodates the
larger size of flexible cable used with portable x-ray apparatus. Other
socket outlets must be provided in the nursing station and general
working area for cleaning equipment etc.

Heating and Ventilation

The heating system should be capable of continuous operation so that
it is available on cold days in the summer. An even temperature is
important in view of the exposure of the patients in an I.T.U. for
observation purposes. Ventilation should preferably be by mechanical
means with suitably placed input and extraction ducts, and air conditioning is desirable, the air being washed, filtered, dried and if
necessary cooled. A hot humid atmosphere in the summer can be
extremely trying both for patients and staff.

Wash basins

Basins should be sufficient in number and properly sited, with either

Design Features

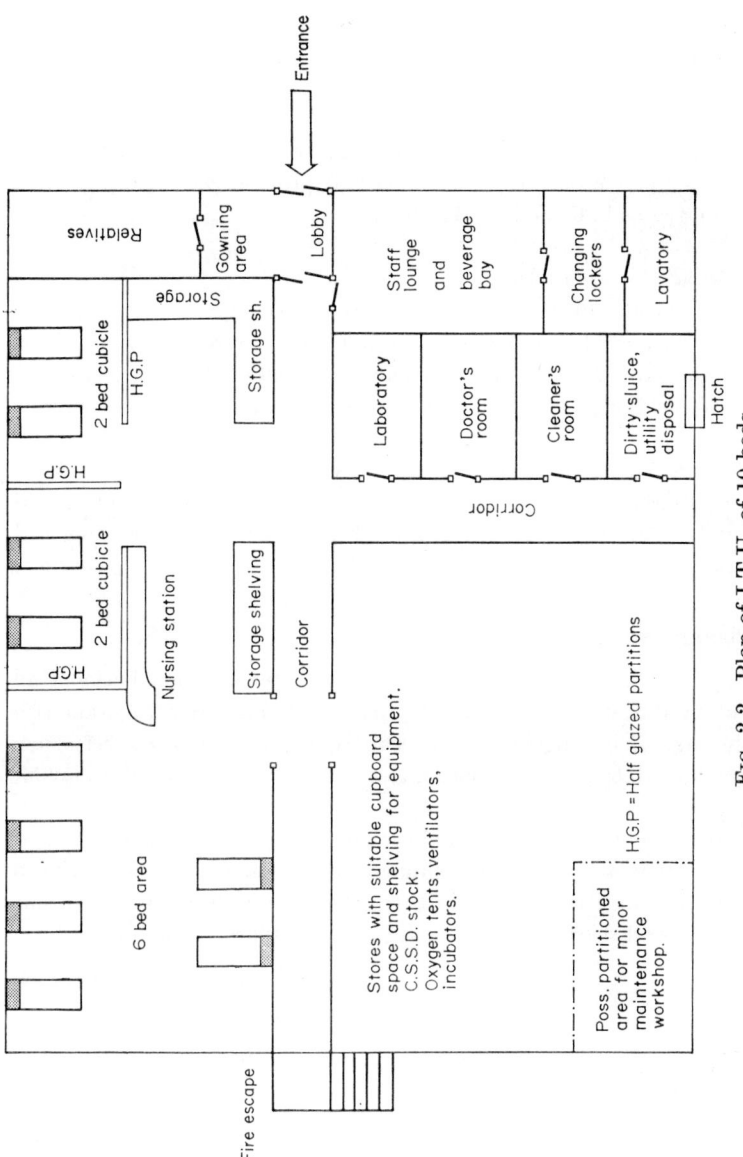

Fig. 2.2 Plan of I.T.U. of 10 beds.

foot-operated or lever-operated taps and a suitable mixing device for hot and cold water.

Telephones

These should be situated at the central nursing station, staff lounge and doctor's room. The telephone will provide the external alarm necessary as indicated in Chapter 18.

Internal Warning Alarm

An emergency button should be situated at each bed station, sounding an alarm audible throughout the whole unit, so that assistance can be summoned quickly. The alarm tone should *not* be the same as the bell notifying the presence of visitors at the entrance lobby of the unit.

Clocks

Large-faced silent-running electric clocks with a centre sweep second hand should be so sited that a clock can be viewed from each bed station.

Planning an I.T.U.

Any I.T.U. should be planned after full consultation between all potential users, and is preferably purpose built. Older hospitals with the large Nightingale type of ward may be able to convert such accommodation by partitions into a suitable unit. A suggested layout is given in Fig. 2.2.

It is important to have windows for natural lighting, in the patient area particularly, as older children subjected entirely to artificial lighting may lose all sense of time. It is also desirable to have some sort of wall decoration (e.g. paintings) to relieve monotony.

FURTHER READING

'Hospital Building Note No. 27: *Intensive Therapy Unit*, H.M.S.O. August, 1970.

CHAPTER

3

Infection, Cross-Infection and Sterilisation

Severely ill patients have an increased susceptibility to infection, and those in an intensive therapy ward are even more at risk as some of the natural barriers to the entry of infection have been breached, for example by the insertion of endotracheal tubes, urethral catheters, intravenous and intra-arterial cannulae. It is almost impossible to manage an endotracheal tube or tracheostomy without the introduction of *some* bacteria, but all possible precautions should be taken during suction. There is also bound to be some stasis of secretions, as an effective cough is impossible, and this will encourage the growth of bacteria. Intravenous cannulae have been shown to be a source of infection, especially if left *in situ* for long periods. Inferior vena caval infusions through a cannula inserted in the groin are particularly hazardous, perhaps because of the proximity of the perineal area. Most severely ill patients receive potent antibiotics, either prophylactically or for established infection. The balance of the commensal bacterial flora in the bowel is upset, and there is a danger of monilial invasion. Small babies are particularly prone to this. The result may be diarrhoea, oral 'thrush', monilial infection of the oesophagus and/or trachea and tracheostomy wounds, skin rashes, or Candida albicans septicaemia.

In spite of precautions, all intensive therapy units tend to have a resident bacterial flora. The sources of infection are many:

Dust
Bacteria are carried in dust, and this may come into the unit through

open windows, it may be carried in as dirt on shoes, or contributed to by particles from bedding and clothing. The bacteria contaminating the dust come from wounds, excreta, apparatus, or, most commonly as droplets from coughing and sneezing on the part of patients, staff, or visitors. Still air is said to be sterile, but in a busy area the air is constantly disturbed, and dust is disseminated throughout. It settles on flat surfaces such as cupboards and floors, and on wounds, open tracheostomies etc. Growth of bacteria is encouraged by a humid atmosphere, and discouraged by desiccation.

Cross-infection
Bacteria may be transferred between patients by the hands and clothing of attending staff. They may originate from wounds, dressings or excreta.

Autogenous
Commensal bacteria in the pharynx and bowel may cause infection in the presence of severe illness.

Water
If left standing, water is rapidly colonised by bacteria, and this constitutes a hazard in humidifiers. Incubators also tend to become a source of infection.

The bacteria most commonly present are Gram-negative bacilli, such as Ps. pyocyanea, E.coli and Klebsiella. Gram-positive organisms such as Staphylococcus aureus and Streptococci also occur, but are a less common cause of infection.

Eradication of infection depends on the awareness of the possibility of infection, and on early detection. Routine sampling should be undertaken as well as more specific sampling when infection is suspected.

Routine sampling of the environment may be by slit samplers or settle plates for the air, and impression plates for bedding etc. Water from humidifiers and incubators, and disinfectant solutions from suction bottles, should be regularly examined. Culture of bacteriological swabs from the nose and throat of attending personnel will help to detect carriers of infection, especially Staphylococcus aureus. Suction catheters from endotracheal or tracheostomy tubes are normally cultured weekly. If bacteria are detected by routine sampling

Infection, Cross-Infection and Sterilisation

it must be determined whether these are pathogenic, although some normally harmless bacteria may become pathogenic in the presence of severe illness. Typing of organisms by the bacteriologist can be of assistance in determining the incidence of cross-infection. Heavy contamination of wound and tracheal swabs or urine does not necessarily mean the presence of infection unless pus cells are also seen.

Specific sampling must be done whenever infection is suspected. It is important that infection is recognised and treated early, but diagnosis may be hindered by the already poor state of the patient. Purulent discharges from the trachea, bladder, wounds etc. should immediately be examined bacteriologically. Continuous monitoring and observation should detect signs of systemic infection, which include elevated temperature, sweating, tachycardia and raised respiratory rate. A differential white blood cell count may also be useful, and blood culture must be done if septicaemia is suspected. Gram-negative septicaemia causes severe shock and has a high mortality rate. Early detection and treatment is important from the point of view of the individual patient, but, also, his infection constitutes a cross-infection hazard to other patients.

Treatment of infection with the appropriate antibiotics should be commenced as soon as possible. Except in specific instances, such as cardiac surgery, it is doubtful if prophylactic antibiotics should be used because the advent of infection may be masked, resistant strains of bacteria produced, and monilial infection may be encouraged.

THE CONTROL OF INFECTION

Airborne bacteria, droplets and dust

A well designed unit with surfaces easy to clean and lacking crevices, will facilitate the control of dust. A mat should be placed at the entrance to remove dirt from shoes. Wet dusting, wet mopping and vacuum cleaning all remove dust without too much disturbance of the air.

Traffic through the unit should be kept to a minimum. It is useful to have a deterrent to easy entry, such as a routine of putting on gowns and overshoes, or an air-lock. Gowns should always be worn over street clothes, but overshoes, although a useful deterrent to entry, probably carry bacteria into the unit. The routine wearing of caps and masks is uncomfortable and unnecessary, and may be frightening to small children but perhaps masks should be worn in the presence of infectious patients, or if the visitor has a cold.

Properly controlled ventilation and air conditioning, with recirculation of filtered air, and control of humidity, will help to remove air-borne bacteria. On the other hand, an enclosed area with no windows may produce psychiatric disturbances in patients and staff.

Cross-infection

Beds should not be too close together, otherwise droplet infection may occur between patients. For meticulous control of cross-infection it is best to have patients in cubicles, but such a system requires a large nursing staff, and it is more practical to keep one or two cubicles for isolation of infectious patients. Bed linen must be changed regularly especially if soiled with secretions. The hands of attendants must of course be washed between procedures and between handling different patients. Hands should not be scrubbed excessively to the point of excoriation as the nurse's skin may thereby become infected and constitute a risk to patients. A mask should be worn for dressing wounds, cutting down on veins, inserting urethral catheters etc.

It may be best to avoid taking the temperature rectally, because of the risk of contaminating the hands with bowel organisms. In small children, however, this is the only practical route for recording 'core' temperature and it may be best for the nurse to wear disposable gloves for the procedure.

Tracheal toilet must be performed with care. Sterile disposable suction catheters must be used, and discarded if contaminated by touching the bed, or the outside of endotracheal connections. The use of disposable sterile plastic gloves reduces the risk of cross-infection, and makes the technique easier. In some units sterile forceps are used to introduce the catheter. A catheter which has been used to aspirate the mouth and nose must *never* be introduced into the trachea.

Apparatus

Suction bottles and chest drainage bottles should be changed and cleaned routinely. Sterile water should be delivered in small bottles to obviate the necessity of leaving larger containers standing open to the air.

Humidifiers, incubators and ventilators constitute a potential reservoir of infection and must be sterilised between use for different patients. It is possible that such equipment should be routinely changed during use on the *same* patient, because it rapidly becomes contaminated by the patient, constituting a source of autogenous infection, and the water may be colonised from the atmosphere. Regular changing of such equipment demands a large reserve store and efficient sterilisation methods.

STERILISATION AND THE SUPPLY OF STERILE EQUIPMENT

In most large hospitals sterile equipment and packs are supplied by a Central Sterile Supply Department. This reduces the work load on the nursing staff, but often means that there is no equipment for sterilising articles on the ward. It is advisable to retain a small electrically operated autoclave for instruments required rapidly.

Packs for dressings, intravenous cutdowns, insertion of chest drains, etc. are supplied, and disposable syringes, needles and catheters are used. The material used to wrap packs must be permeable to the sterilising agent and is usually paper, or cloth or a combination of the two. Plastic film is used for endotracheal tubes and some disposable equipment. Glassware, such as suction bottles, is often sterilised by heat in metal containers. Whatever material is used for packs, it must be impermeable to dust and bacteria when the packs are in store. Instruments must be washed after use, before being returned to the C.S.S.D. Very contaminated articles should be soaked in disinfectant solution before being washed and sterilised, to protect the handler. It is important to remove débris before sterilisation, which may otherwise be inefficient.

The method of sterilisation depends on the material to be sterilised and the procedure available.

Heat

Moist heat under pressure is the method of choice, provided the equipment can withstand it. Autoclaving is used for packs, instruments, dressings, endotracheal tubes (rubber) and rubber ventilator tubing. Some plastic ventilator tubing will also withstand heat. Dry heat in a hot air oven is used for glassware and some delicate instruments. Boiling may be used to sterilise the metal parts of respirators and anaesthetic equipment.

Gamma irradiation
Disposable plastic syringes, needles, catheters, endotracheal tubes and plastic tubing are sterilised by this method. Some hospitals have access to this procedure for non-disposable equipment. It should be noted that material sterilised originally in this way must not later be exposed to ethylene oxide, as toxic products are formed.

Ethylene oxide
This gas is toxic and precautions to protect personnel must be strict. The gas is very expensive. Materials to be sterilised should first be cleaned and dried. As much air as possible should be evacuated from the container before the gas is admitted, in order to improve contact and reduce explosion risks.

Ethylene oxide can be used to sterilise electrical apparatus, heart-lung machines (but not the tubing), pacemakers, cardiac catheters, some needles, and also ventilators and incubators. After exposure to the gas the equipment should be aerated for 12 hours at 50°C or allowed to stand at room temperature for at least 48 hours, to allow escape of the gas, otherwise tissue irritation may occur.

Soaking in antiseptic solutions
This may be used as a preliminary method of cleaning, or for definitive sterilisation of such articles as ventilator tubing, endotracheal connectors, and storage of forceps, scissors etc. Many solutions are in use, some more effective than others. Aqueous chlorhexidine however has been shown to support the growth of Ps. pyocyanea. Probably the most effective solution is 'Cidex'* (activated dialdehyde), but it is very expensive.

Fumigation with formaldehyde vapour
This can be used for incubators, ventilators, suction apparatus etc. It should be followed by ammonia, to neutralise the formaldehyde, and the apparatus well aerated afterwards.

Ventilators
A recent method of sterilising ventilators uses an ultrasonic nebuliser, and a closed ventilator circuit. Alcohol may be used, but is very explosive with air, and should be used with 100 per cent nitrogen. Less explosive, and claimed to be effective, is hydrogen peroxide.

* Manufactured by Arbrook Limited, Edinburgh.

CHAPTER

4

Fluid, Electrolyte and Metabolic Balance

Surgical stress and severe disease lead to extensive and often prolonged changes which modify the nutritional requirements of the patient.

The materials required by the body can be divided into two groups:
1. Obligatory substances entering into the structure of the body, namely water, electrolytes, vitamins, and proteins, which are necessary for tissue synthesis.
2. Energy-providing substances, namely carbohydrates, fats and proteins.

WATER

Body water is distributed between two compartments of the body, namely, intracellular and extracellular, but there is a continuous process of inter-change from one to the other. The extracellular water is further subdivided into that which is present in the blood (the vascular compartment) and that which surrounds the cells in the tissues (the interstitial compartment).

Whereas the composition of plasma reflects fairly well the state of the interstitial fluid, it does not indicate the conditions prevailing within the cells, so that plasma electrolyte estimations may be fairly normal in the presence of severe intracellular disturbances.

The total body water content represents a balance between intake (as fluids, and from oxidation of foods) and output (losses from the skin, the lungs, the gastrointestinal tract and the kidneys). Only a small proportion of the body's need for water is supplied by oxidation processes.

Proportional to its size the infant has a greater body water content than the child, and the child more than the adult. Approximate values are given in Table 4.1.

Table 4.1 Body water distribution expressed as percentage of body weight in Kg.

Compartment	0–1 month	1 month–1 year	1–12 years
Intracellular	45	45	45
Extracellular	30	25	20
Total Body Water	75	70	65

Note that with age, change occurs in the *extracellular compartment*, but at all ages plasma forms about 5 per cent of body weight (8 per cent of body weight represents the blood volume). The main difference with age therefore is in the amount of interstitial fluid.

It is important to realise that under normal conditions the balance of sodium and water in the body is closely interrelated and this will be considered later. Water requirements decrease as the child gets older, as shown in Table 4.2.

Table 4.2 Normal water requirements.

Age in Years	Water Requirement ml/Kg of body weight
0–1	150
1–3	100
3–6	90
7+	70

During the first week of life the need for water is less than 150 ml/Kg and is best calculated as a proportion for age; thus on the first day of life the requirement would be $1/7 \times 150$ ml/Kg, on the fourth day it would be $4/7 \times 150$ ml/Kg and so on.

Premature infants of low birth weight require more fluid than those of normal size, and requirements should be based on 200 ml/Kg body weight.

SODIUM

This is primarily an extracellular ion, and is retained in the body in solution as sodium chloride. Total body sodium amounts to about

Fluid, Electrolyte and Metabolic Balance

58 mEq/Kg of body weight, and slightly less than half of this is contained in the bones. Under normal circumstances the dietary intake shows fairly wide variations, and the loss of sodium in sweat is also variable. The kidney is the chief organ regulating the body sodium level. Active reabsorption of filtered sodium ions occurs in the proximal part of the renal tubules, a process for which the hormone aldosterone, secreted by the adrenal cortex, is essential. Thus adrenocortical stimulation will cause sodium (and therefore water) retention, while drugs such as spironolactone block the effect of aldosterone and thus promote sodium (and therefore water) loss. During sodium reabsorption water is also reabsorbed *passively*. Lower down the renal tubules water reabsorption can occur, *actively*, a process which is affected by the antidiuretic hormone (ADH) produced by the pituitary. ADH production is inhibited by the oral intake of large quantities of water or intravenous infusion of hypotonic saline or isotonic glucose solution, and the specific gravity of the urine falls. Dehydration, on the other hand, stimulates ADH production and body water is conserved, so that urine of high specific gravity is voided.

Sodium balance depends on intake versus losses. The normal plasma range is 136–145 mEq/L and the approximate daily requirement (in the absence of abnormal losses) is shown in Table 4.3.

Table 4.3 Maintenance sodium requirements.

Age in Years	Sodium mEq/Kg of body weight
0–1	2·5
1–3	2·5
3–6	2·0
7–12	1·5

Hyponatraemia

A low *serum* sodium may be found in true sodium depletion, primary water overload, cardiac failure, hypoproteinaemia, inappropiate secretion of antidiuretic hormone, and in the 'sick cell' syndrome.

True sodium depletion occurs when there has been excessive salt loss from the alimentary tract, or a failure by the kidneys to retain sodium, and therefore indicates a greater loss of sodium relative to water, *or* water replacement which has exceeded that of sodium. It may therefore *result* from incorrect replacement therapy. The sodium required to correct a deficit can be calculated from the formula:

Sodium mEq = (140 − serum sodium mEq/L) × Total body water as per cent of body weight in Kg, taking 140 as the 'normal' serum sodium level.

Primary water overload results from an excess of water intake over sodium, or defective excretion of water. In the paediatric age group this is most likely to follow the infusion of excess hypotonic solutions and solutions containing no sodium. It results in cellular overhydration and cerebral oedema, causing unconsciousness and convulsions. Urgent treatment, involving the use of hypertonic saline, and perhaps mannitol to promote a diuresis, is necessary to avoid permanent brain damage.

In cardiac failure hyponatraemia is not uncommon. However, hyponatraemia in the presence of systemic venous oedema and a raised central venous pressure does not indicate salt depletion, but means that the total body sodium is raised. The hyponatraemia results from inadequate excretion of water, and, if renal function is not impaired, will respond to osmotic diuretics. A similar state can result from impaired osmolarity in hypoproteinaemia.

In meningitis, certain cerebral tumours, encephalitis and head injuries, there may be excessive production of antidiuretic hormone, associated with a block of aldosterone production, so that there is retention and expansion of total body water with excessive sodium losses.

Impaired function of the 'sodium pump' can occur in a variety of pathological states, with a loss of sodium ions from the extracellular fluid into the cells, and a consequent migration of potassium from the cells into the extracellular compartment. This is the so-called 'sick cell' syndrome, and the ionic pump mechanism of the cell membrane is influenced by the insulin secretion of the pancreas. Thus in diabetic coma the serum sodium is low and the potassium is high, a state which reverts to normal after insulin therapy and the correction of the metabolic acidosis.

Hypernatraemia

This usually arises from inadequate water intake despite continuing water excretion, either because of high solute loads, or due to defective tubular reabsorption of water. It may arise where there are high losses of water other than urinary. As with hyponatraemia, there may be low, normal or high total body sodium levels.

Hypernatraemia due to sodium overloading is accompanied usually by an expanded extracellular compartment, but when due to water deficit the extracellular fluid is reduced and there are clinical signs of dehydration. The water deficit can be calculated approximately from the formula.

$$\text{Water deficit in litres} = \left(1 - \frac{\text{serum sodium mEq/L}}{140}\right) \times \text{total body water as per cent of body weight in Kg}$$

CHLORIDE

Chloride ions are present in both the extracellular and intracellular compartments, and in combination with sodium play an essential part in water balance, as well as in acid/base regulation. Dietary intake is almost exclusively as sodium chloride, and in general terms renal handling and sweat loss of chloride follow the same patterns as sodium. In acid/base disturbances chloride plays a special part by virtue of its exchange with bicarbonate ion (the chloride shift q.v. Chapter 5) and the usual proportions of chloride and bicarbonate associated with sodium may not be found, either in the blood or in the urine.

It must be stressed that chloride and sodium are not present in plasma in equal amounts; the normal plasma range of chloride is 96–108 mEq/L and the relationship of chloride to sodium is shown by the formula.

Sodium mEq/L = Chloride mEq/L + Bicarbonate mEq/L + 10.

Abnormalities of sodium metabolism are generally accompanied by abnormalities of chloride. Thus sodium losses in diarrhoea, profuse sweating, adrenogenital syndrome, Waterhouse-Friderichsen syndrome etc., are accompanied by a corresponding chloride deficit, but predominant chloride loss can occur as in the vomiting of pyloric obstruction.

POTASSIUM

This is primarily the cation for maintaining the correct pH of intracellular fluid, but it is also a very important constituent of the extracellular fluid since it influences muscle activity, notably that of cardiac muscle. All cellular activities involving electrical changes (muscle contraction and the conduction of nerve impulses) are dependent on the gradients of potassium and sodium ions across cell membranes. It is important to remember the disproportion of potassium ions between the intracellular compartment and extracellular fluid, the proportion being about 10:1. Thus relatively small shifts from the intracellular compartment can cause large changes in the extracellular fluid.

A further important concept is the transfer of glucose and potassium from the extracellular fluid across the cell membrane and into the cell, a process which is controlled by insulin. Thus in diabetic coma the hyperglycaemia is frequently accompanied by hyperkalaemia; treatment by insulin not only lowers the blood sugar but may also reduce the serum potassium to dangerously low levels by causing potassium ions to be driven into the cells.

The kidney is the main organ for potassium excretion and the total body potassium depends on the balance struck between intake and output. Adrenocortical stimulation, in contrast to what happens with sodium, increases the renal loss of potassium. Potassium losses are excessive where tissue breakdown occurs, and where lower renal tubule reabsorprion of water is impaired, (for example, certain renal diseases, or the use of diuretics which block tubular reabsorption).

Potassium is an essential ion required for protein reconstruction and tissue synthesis. This is important in the anabolic phase of repair after surgery or the healing of disease processes, and it has been estimated that a loss of 5 Kg of muscle proteins requires 600 mEq of potassium together with the necessary protein nitrogen for its replacement.

Potassium depletion tends to produce a metabolic alkalosis and conversely an alkalosis predisposes to hypokalaemia. Whenever an alkalosis proves resistant to theoretically adequate corrective measures, the possibility of potassium deficiency must be considered. In these cases, usually the urine is paradoxically acid and not alkaline.

The normal plasma range is 3·5–5·5 mEq/L and the approximate daily requirement is shown in Table 4.4. It is important to remember that considerable deficits of total body potassium may exist with little or no fall in serum levels.

Fluid, Electrolyte and Metabolic Balance

Table 4.4 Maintenance potassium requirements.

Age in Years	Potassium mEq/Kg of body weight
0–1	2·5
1–3	2·5
3–6	2·0
7–12	1·5

Hypokalaemia

Since sodium is an extracellular ion, salt and water balance is fairly easy to assess and control. Potassium balance depends on the distribution of potassium between the cells and the extracellular compartment, and serum levels are almost useless as a means of estimating total body potassium. Moreover, the serum potassium can change relatively rapidly, owing to translocation between the extracellular and intracellular compartments.

Total body potassium may be moderately depleted without much effect on serum levels, but when severe deficiency is present the serum potassium is usually below 3·5 mEq/L and there is a metabolic alkalosis with a standard bicarbonate greater than 31 mEq/L, and the serum chloride is low. Potassium depletion may be concealed in the presence of dehydration and sodium loss, and indeed the serum level may then be high; only when the deficit of the extracellular compartment has been repaired does the serum show hypokalaemia. Excess potassium loss occurs usually either from the gastro-intestinal tract, or in the urine (for example, patients who have renal disease, or who are receiving adrenocortical stimulating steroids, or diuretics).

Potassium depletion causes dysfunction of cardiac, skeletal and smooth muscle. Thus in paralytic ileus there is a loss of potassium into the lumen of the distended alimentary tract, and the potassium deficit contributes to the ileus. Cardiac manifestations of hypokalaemia include prolongation of the Q–T interval, a decrease in height of the T waves, which may become inverted, and S–T segment depression. Arrhythmias may occur—typically paroxysmal atrial tachycardia and variable atrio-ventricular block. It must be emphasised that the cardiac features are not usually seen *early* in potassium depletion and may take up to 48 hours to appear. It is important to realise that a potassium deficit causes an increased sensitivity to digitalis so that toxic effects can appear. The skeletal effects include muscular weakness and flaccid paralysis. A chronic hypokalaemic state causes impaired renal function with inability to conserve water even when there is inadequate water intake, so that excessive amounts of urine are passed and the patient becomes thirsty.

Hyperkalaemia

This may arise because of the inability of the cell membrane to prevent loss of potassium ions into the extracellular space following ischaemia, trauma, anoxia or acidosis (stored blood may contain very high amounts of free potassium ions in the plasma: this is of practical importance when blood transfusion is being used, particularly if large volumes are involved, as the potassium-calcium balance can be disturbed, resulting in impaired cardiac function or death).

Hyperkalaemia may also occur due to excessive oral or parenteral intake, when the total body potassium can rise. Whatever it is due to, it is always much more serious when renal function is impaired and urinary output is low.

Toxic effects of potassium are most serious in relation to cardiac action. The earliest change, occurring with a mild to moderate increase of serum potassium, is peaking of the T waves. With increasing levels the QRS complex becomes spread out and the P–R interval is prolonged, indicating increased conduction time in the myocardium. Severe elevation of potassium causes a 'sine wave' appearance due to spreading out of the QRS complex, tenting of the T wave and a curved depression of the S–T segment; this is a pre-fatal electrocardiographic appearance and can progress rapidly to complete heart block and ventricular fibrillation.

It must be stressed that, as with hypokalaemia, the electrocardiographic changes are not precise, and indeed high potassium levels in the presence of normal sodium may cause no cardiac disturbance. Conversely, hyponatraemia and hypocalcaemia will aggravate the effects of hyperkalaemia.

CALCIUM AND MAGNESIUM

These two cations are considered together as they both have an effect on cell membrane permeability. About 99 per cent of the body's calcium is present in the skeleton, and the remainder is in the extracellular fluid; it is both protein-bound and ionized in the plasma, the

Fluid, Electrolyte and Metabolic Balance

extent of ionization being influenced by acid-base balance. Ionized calcium is increased in acidosis and decreased in alkalosis. Bound calcium is mainly linked to albumin so that there is a direct relation between the level of serum albumin and serum calcium. Calcium metabolism is affected by renal handling, this being dependent on parathyroid hormone which favours increased tubular reabsorption of calcium ions, while probably depressing tubular reabsorption of phosphate. The total serum calcium depends on the amount of dietary calcium which is absorbed from the intestine together with the amount reabsorbed from the renal tubules, and on the loss in the urine and by deposition in the skeleton. Parathyroid hormone also promotes intestinal absorption and the mobilisation of calcium from bone. Secretion of the hormone is stimulated by a fall in the serum ionized calcium. The normal plasma level is 4·5–5·8 mEq/L.

Magnesium also exists in a protein-bound and ionized form in the plasma. About 70 per cent of body magnesium is combined with calcium and phosphate in the skeleton, and the remainder is contained in the soft-tissues and body fluids. Whole blood contains 1·7–3·4 mEq/L whereas plasma contains less than half this amount, showing that there is a relatively greater intracellular content. Muscle contains about 21–23 mg/100 gm, and it may function as an activator for the enzymes of the glycolytic systems of carbohydrate metabolism. About ten times the quantity of magnesium contained in extracellular fluid is present in the cells, a differential distribution which is comparable with that found in the case of potassium ion.

It has been suggested that calcium and magnesium ions have a mutually antagonistic effect. It has been shown experimentally that intravenous injection of magnesium salts produces anaesthesia and paralysis of voluntary muscles, which can be reversed by injection of a corresponding amount of calcium.

A fall of ionized calcium leads to blood coagulation defects, impaired cardiac function, impaired cell membrane permeability and neuromuscular irritability. The latter may become manifest as tetany, and this is believed to involve complex ionic relationships, of which the determinant factor is a fall in the ratio:

$$\frac{Ca^{++} + Mg^{++} + H^+}{Na^+ + K^+}$$

In neonatal tetany due to hypocalcaemia it is sometimes found that the hyperirritable state persists despite adequately increased calcium intake, and some of these patients respond to magnesium given in addition.

Magnesium excess causes central nervous system depression with loss of tendon reflexes and the production of drowsiness progressing to coma. The heart responds by a slowing of rate and increased conduction time through the conducting tissue and myocardium.

THE EXTRACELLULAR FLUID

Clinically, the volume of the extracellular fluid is assessed somewhat crudely by such criteria as the state of the skin and subcutaneous tissues, and the state of the circulation. Laboratory investigations which may be helpful are the haematocrit, and measurement of blood and plasma volume.

Serial haematocrit determinations are useful in assessing the correction of fluid deficits, but the limitations of this must be recognised. The packed cell volume may be *normal* in an anaemic but fluid depleted patient, and it may be *low* merely as a result of anaemia. The picture is further complicated if *blood* loss is present in addition to fluid and electrolyte imbalance, and also when blood transfusion is being used. Serial haematocrits are of *some* value in monitoring replacement therapy of losses from the vascular compartment due to haemorrhage.

Equipment used for measuring blood volume employs such materials as radioactive chromium-labelled red cells, or isotopically-labelled albumin. In order to be accurate the indicator must mix thoroughly with the plasma. A further limitation of the technique is that it measures the blood volume *at the time*, and to be of value serial measurements have to be made. Comparison of the measured blood volume with the estimated 'normal' can lead to serious errors in management.

Depletion of extracellular fluid results in impaired circulation and hypotension, with tachycardia, peripheral vasoconstriction and laxity of the subcutaneous tissues. Severe depletion can cause lethargy, mental confusion and eventually death. Over-expansion of the extracellular compartment produces a rise of central venous pressure, peripheral oedema and pulmonary oedema. A severe overload of the compartment can cause cerebral confusion and convulsions.

In view of the difficulty of clinical assessment of the state of the

Fluid, Electrolyte and Metabolic Balance

extracellular compartment, a therapeutic trial may be necessary in order to resolve a particular problem, isotonic electrolyte solution being adminstered intravenously while the central venous pressure is carefully monitored. When this begins to rise above the upper limit of normal it can be assumed that the extracellular compartment is restored to a normal volume, (this presumes that the patient does not have co-existing cardiovascular disease with incipient or actual congestive failure).

DISTURBANCES OF WATER AND ELECTROLYTES

Estimation of losses of fluid and electrolyte can be extremely difficult, and there are no simple investigations available to determine them. Body weight *changes* are a valuable guide to the adequacy of therapy, *but* if a child is seen in whom the pre-dehydration weight is not known, the dehydrated weight can only give an approximate guide to the extent of the fluid loss by comparison with the estimated 'normal' weight for his age and size. Clinical assessment is still the best way of making the first appraisal of the state of the body fluids.

In *mild* dehydration the child is irritable and thirsty, with a dry tongue and mouth. The eyes are slightly sunken but bright, and the face is flushed and warm. This degree of fluid loss corresponds to a deficit of 15 per cent of extracellular fluid. (See Table 4.1).

Moderate dehydration, amounting to a 22·5 per cent loss of extracellular fluid, is evidenced by restlessness, with an anxious, alert expression. There is extreme thirst and dryness of the mouth and tongue. The eyes are very sunken, and the fontanelle, in the case of infants, is depressed. The urine output is low, and the child is febrile with a rapid pulse. Skin elasticity is poor.

In *severe* dehydration the child is apathetic and unresponsive or unconscious. There is generalized hypotonia, the eyes are staring and sunken, and the fontanelle if still open is very depressed. The mouth is extremely dry, and circulatory collapse is evidenced by a feeble, thready, rapid pulse with cold, cyanosed extremities. This corresponds to a deficit of 30 per cent of extracellular fluid.

When dealing with infants confusion has arisen because it has been thought in the past that the infant's kidney is unable to handle sodium as effectively as can the adult's. Recent work, however, suggests that the infant's kidney fails to retain sodium even in the presence of hyponatraemia. Although in many instances dehydration involves the loss of water and sodium in a proportional manner—*isotonic dehydration*—so that fairly normal serum sodium levels may be found, the replacement of fluid loss by water alone as dextrose solutions would have the possibility of causing a primary water overload, and it must be remembered that in isotonic dehydration the *total* body sodium is depleted so that sodium must also be given in the repair schedule.

If an infant has lost large quantities of water but little sodium—*hypernatraemic dehydration*, with a higher than normal serum sodium—he will appear deceptively well hydrated with relatively little peripheral circulatory failure and little impairment of skin elasticity, as the vascular compartment is not markedly contracted.

Dehydration associated with a disproportionately large sodium loss—*hyponatraemic dehydration*—shows low serum sodium levels.

When assessing sodium loss it must be emphasized that, although sodium is normally confined to the extracellular compartment, its osmotic effect is distributed throughout all the body fluids. Thus addition of sodium to the extracellular fluid will increase its osmolarity resulting in a withdrawal of fluid from the cells. Therefore, although water deficit estimation and replacement is based on consideration of the *extracellular fluid*, sodium requirements are based on *total body water* estimations.

If fluid and electrolytes are being taken by mouth in the normal diet, good renal function is present and there are no abnormal losses, then the body is capable of excellent control both of fluid and electrolyte balance. However, when metabolic processes have been disturbed as a result of disease or trauma, and abnormal losses of fluid and electrolytes occur, imbalance can be produced by illconsidered intravenous administration of fluid and electrolyte solutions.

The basis of fluid and electrolyte therapy

Children receiving parenteral fluids *must* be re-evaluated at frequent intervals, and a careful reassessment made every twenty-four hours. When correcting severe electrolyte disturbances it is essential to carry out periodic serum electrolyte estimations which can be done on capillary blood, if necessary every few hours. Daily weight records provide the best guide to fluctuations in hydration. Intake and out-

Fluid, Electrolyte and Metabolic Balance

put records must be kept *in detail*, and *all* losses must be measured accurately. Urine volumes, with measurement of the twenty-four hours excretion of electrolytes and urea are necessary recordings, and it is important to note whether the urine is pale and dilute, or dark and concentrated, and to measure the specific gravity of the various amounts after they have been voided. Losses from various parts of the alimentary tract should be recorded, and to be meticulous the electrolyte loss from these routes should be measured. However, extra renal losses can be estimated fairly accurately by measuring the twenty-four hour volume loss and calculating from data given in Table 4.5.

Table 4.5 Electrolyte content of Alimentary Fluids mEq/L.

Alimentary Fluid	Hydrogen ion	Sodium	Potassium	Bicarbonate	Chloride
Saliva	—	15–20	20–30	20	20
Gastric juice	40–60	20–80	5–20	—	100–150
Bile	—	120–140	5–15	30–50	80–120
Pancreatic juices	—	120–140	5–15	70–110	40–80
Small intestine	—	100–140	5–15	20–40	90–130

Fluid and electrolyte replacement falls into three subdivisions: the provision of maintenance requirements, the repair of existing deficits, and the provision for continuing losses. The last of these requires some amplification. Just as blood loss should be replaced *as it occurs*, so fluid and electrolyte loss (for example, aspiration of large amounts of gastric secretion through a Ryle's tube) should be made good every few hours and one should not wait for a deficit to build up which would require correction in the next twenty-four hours régime. It is important, therefore, to have frequent reappraisal of the patient, both clinically and biochemically.

It is preferable in treating cases of dehydration to avoid the use of polyionic infusion solutions such as Hartman's since these rarely provide electrolytes in the proportions required by the individual patient. Moreover, if the patient is acidotic with a low standard bicarbonate, the administration of lactate provides only a slow correction since it has to be metabolized to bicarbonate. However, such infusions are of use in the older child in order to avoid the administration of too much chloride ion, as may occur with saline infusions, causing metabolic acidosis.

Suitable infusion solutions are given in Table 4.6.

Table 4.6 Infusion solutions supplied in 500 ml bottles.

Solution	Sodium mEq/L	Chloride mEq/L	Potassium mEq/L
0·9% sodium chloride with or without 5% dextrose	154	154	—
0·18% sodium chloride with 4·3% dextrose	30·8	30·8	—
5% or 10% dextrose	—	—	—
5% or 10% laevulose	—	—	—
M/6 sodium lactate	167	—	—
M/6 ammonium chloride	—	170	—
Hartman's (Ringer-Lactate)	130	104	4
2N saline	308	308	—
50% dextrose	—	—	—
20% mannitol	—	—	—

In addition to these certain ampoules should be available as shown in Table 4.7.

Table 4.7 Supplementary solutions in fluid and electrolyte therapy.

Ampoules	Electrolyte content
20 ml of 8·4% sodium bicarbonate in water	1 ml contains 1 mEq of bicarbonate and 1 mEq of sodium
5 ml containing 0·15 gm of potassium chloride in water	Total content 2 mEq of potassium and 2 mEq of chloride
5 ml containing 1·0 gm of potassium chloride in water	Total content 13 mEq of potassium and 13 mEq of chloride
10 ml of 10% calcium gluconate	0·45 mEq of calcium per ml
5 ml of 10% calcium chloride	0·9 mEq of calcium per ml

These solutions require some explanation. 0·9 per cent (normal) saline, is a truly isotonic solution, whereas combined with 5 per cent dextrose it is hypertonic and will cause some expansion of the extracellular compartment; this possible disadvantage may be offset by the provision of calories in the dextrose-saline version. Hypertonic solution such as 10 per cent dextrose and 10 per cent laevulose are not of importance in the context of fluid and electrolyte maintenance and repair, but may be useful as part of the schedule designed to provide energy (q.v. later).

Very hypertonic solutions such as 50 per cent dextrose are useful if cellular overhydration is present, and cause a translocation of water

Fluid, Electrolyte and Metabolic Balance

from the intracellular compartment to the extracellular fluid, but such osmotic transfer of water is probably better accomplished by infusion of 20 per cent mannitol (in a dose of 1 gm/Kg of body weight), which has the advantage of increasing renal blood flow and glomerular filtration.

Hypertonic saline (2N and sometimes 4N) is used where sodium is required as a result of primary water overload in the presence of salt depletion, resulting in cerebral cellular overhydration and convulsions. The return to normal plasma osmolarity often results in rapid improvement.

M/6 sodium lactate and M/6 ammonium chloride are sometimes employed to correct metabolic acidosis and alkalosis respectively, the amount used being based on the carbon dioxide combining power (normal 20–27 mEq/L). Thus 4 ml/Kg of body weight of M/6 sodium lactate raises the carbon dioxide combining power by 1 mEq/L while 2 ml/Kg of body weight of M/6 ammonium chloride lowers the carbon dioxide combining power by 1 mEq/L. As explained in Chapter 5. metabolic acidosis is more usually treated nowadays by intravenous injection of 8·4 per cent sodium bicarbonate solution based on the base deficit estimated by the Astrup technique, and indeed, since lactate requires metabolising to bicarbonate before it becomes available the direct provision of bicarbonate ions seems more logical.

It is not often that metabolic alkalosis requires infusion of chloride ions, as this is usually a self correcting condition, given good renal function and provided the cause of the alkalosis is dealt with. If chloride ions are needed M/6 ammonium chloride can be infused in the appropriate volume to provide the calculated amount of chloride according to the formula:

Chloride mEq. = Base excess (Bicarbonate) mEq/L × 0·3
× body weight in Kg

this being the correction according to the volume of extracellular fluid, and therefore an undercorrection since no account is taken of the intracellular chloride and bicarbonate.

Potassium requirements are best provided as definite amounts to be added to the infusion solutions and measured doses are therefore provided in ampoules. As a rule potassium administration should not exceed 3 mEq/Kg of body weight in 24 hours in the case of infants, or 2 mEq/Kg of body weight in children over one year, if given intravenously, and indeed it is preferable to administer potassium chloride orally whenever possible. In *no case* should the concentration of potassium infused exceed a concentration of 40 mEq/L, as toxic effects can be produced. Hyperkalaemia is an emergency, which should be treated by withholding further potassium administration by all routes, and giving calcium gluconate 10 per cent solution intravenously in a dose of 3 ml/Kg of body weight. As calcium gluconate contains only a small proportion of ionized calcium, in an extreme emergency (e.g. cardiac arrest) calcium chloride 10 per cent solution diluted with normal saline may be given intravenously *very cautiously* with electrocardiographic monitoring, the injection being stopped if the heart rate begins to slow. An additional measure is the intravenous administration of 10 per cent dextrose solution, 10 ml/Kg of body weight, together with 1 unit of soluble insulin for every 5 gm of dextrose to be infused, mixed in with the solution. Resonium A (a cation sodium exchange resin) can be given by gastric tube in a mucilage suspension, in a total dose of 1·25 gm/Kg of body weight in 24 hours, divided into three eight hourly quantities.

In designing a schedule for the individual patient, fluid and electrolyte requirements must be calculated to account for maintenance needs, existing deficits or excesses, and continuing losses. In addition, consideration must be given to the supply of calories to the body.

ENERGY REQUIREMENTS OF THE BODY

The metabolic processes of the body have two aspects requiring consideration: the catabolic phase involving the breakdown of complex molecules with the release of chemical energy, and the anabolic phase whereby chemical energy is stored and complex molecules are synthesized from simple ones. Overall metabolism involves both of these processes, and according to the first law of thermodynamics 'energy can neither be created nor destroyed'. Just as we consider a balance of fluid input and output, so we can consider an energy balance.

Energy and the fuel values of food are most conveniently measured in terms of calories (a calorie being the amount of heat required to raise the temperature of 1 gm of water from 15°C to 16°C). Since this is a small quantity the energy values in metabolic processes are expressed in terms of the kilocalorie or Calorie (equal to 1,000 calories).

Energy in the body is derived ultimately from the chemical energy of food, and the major output by the body is in the form of heat. Chemical energy is required for the metabolic processes in the cells, electrical energy is produced by muscular contraction and neural activity, and mechanical energy is necessary for locomotion etc.

According to the first law of thermodynamics, therefore, energy input of the body must equal its output. Expressed in another way we can say:

Chemical energy of food=Heat energy+work energy+stored chemical energy.

In the fasting patient there is no input of energy from food, so that all energy requirements must be provided from the stored chemical energy. This can only be released by the catabolic phase of breakdown of molecules of stored fat and carbohydrates, and muscle protein, so that wasting occurs.

Carbohydrates furnish about 4 Cals/gm and the daily intake should equal the amount stored in the body. Excess intake is converted to fat. Carbohydrates form the first and most efficient source of energy for vital processes, and a minimum of 5 gm of carbohydrate per 100 Cal of the total diet is required to prevent ketosis. About 70 per cent of the normal Calorie requirement should be provided as carbohydrate.

Dietary fat yields 9 Cals/gm, and, as a form of storage of energy in the body, fat has more than twice the value of carbohydrate or protein. The fat intake is necessary as a supply of 'essential' fatty acids—linoleic and arachidonic—which are unsaturated and exert important effects on lipid metabolism in man. 20 per cent of total Calorie requirement should be in the form of fat.

Proteins provide about 4 Cals/gm, and one sixth of the total weight of protein is present as nitrogen. The basic requirement of nitrogen for the body is 0·1 gm/Kg of body weight (0·6 gm proteins/Kg). The protein requirement is greatly increased in conditions involving increased metabolism (e.g. fever), after destruction of tissue, and during growth. Tissue protein undergoes a process of continual breakdown and resynthesis, and this protein turnover means that nitrogen intake should balance nitrogen loss. Dietary protein is necessary to provide certain essential aminoacids in the laevo-form required for protein synthesis (trytophan, phenylalanine, lysine, threonine, valine, methionine, leucine and iso-leucine).

Although the energy provided by food can be measured outside the body by simple combustion and gives the values stated above, it is found that when used in the body *more* Calories are liberated. Thus 25 gm of protein provide not 100 Cals but 130 Cals, a 100 Cal portion of fat yields in fact 113 Cals, and a 100 Cal portion of carbohydrate 105 Cals. This extra heat production of food elements when used in the body, is referred to as the *specific dynamic action*, and allowance for this has to be made when assessing overall Calorie requirements, which must also allow for Calorie loss in the excreta, while provision must also be made for bodily activity and growth.

The *normal* Calorie requirements are shown for various ages in Table 4.8.

Table 4.8 Calorie requirements for age and body weight.

Age	Cals/Kg
Newborn	110
¼–1 year	100
1–3 years	90
3–6 years	80
7+ years	70

It is important to note that relative to its size the infant's energy requirement is much greater than the adult's. Moreover, the requirement in disease may be much greater than the normal values.

The Basis of Parenteral Nutrition

Given alimentary feeding with good renal function and a balanced diet there is no problem in maintaining adequate nutrition in most patients. However, when disease or trauma cause interference with normal absorptive processes intravenous feeding will be required. This can pose serious difficulties, particularly in infancy, compared with adults. Not the least of these is the difficulty of maintaining an intravenous infusion patent when cannulae are necessarily small and flow rates low, and it has been suggested that a constant infusion pump should be employed. A further risk is that of bacterial and fungal infections during prolonged intravenous therapy. Wherever possible infusion should be set up by percutaneous indwelling cannulae inserted by puncture, rather than by 'cutting down' and sacrificing a peripheral vein, and in infants scalp vein infusion needles are extremely useful.

Fluid, Electrolyte and Metabolic Balance

Whereas normally vitamin supplements are not necessary if a balanced diet is taken by mouth (although infants of course require added vitamins A, D, and C), patients with disease states receiving broad spectrum antibiotic therapy also require additional vitamin intake by injection. Water soluble vitamins can be added to the infusion solutions.

In assessing the requirements for parenteral therapy in the individual patient an estimate must be made of water, electrolyte and energy needs. In order to 'spare' nitrogen in the body it is advisable to aim at a positive balance of intake over output, both of which can be measured. In order to utilize nitrogen properly an adequate Calorie intake in terms of carbohydrate and fat is essential, ideally being 200 Cals/gm of nitrogen infused.

Parenteral nutrition does not mean the haphazard administration of sugar and salt solutions, but the meticulous construction of a schedule designed to provide the fluid, electrolyte and Calories the patient requires, bearing in mind that the latter are greatly increased as a result of disease, with particular reference to the nitrogen component.

Intravenous infusion should therefore provide a source of essential amino acids and also fat, in addition to readily available Calories as carbohydrate. Suitable infusions are shown in Table 4.9.

Aminosol is a dialyzed, enzymatic protein hydrolysate and has the advantage of providing the essential aminoacids in the laevo-form. 'Intralipid' consists of an emulsion of soya bean oil, with egg yolk phosphatides and glycerol in distilled water; it must *not* be given in excess of 2 gm of fat/Kg of body weight in 24 hours (i.e. 10 ml of 20 per cent 'Intralipid'/Kg), and must *not* be allowed to mix with saline otherwise the fine emulsion 'cracks' into larger fat globules. There is some evidence to suggest that both intravenous fat and aminoacid are better utilized by the body if administered *together* through a Y-tube.

Examples of suitable schedules for varying problems will now be given.

Example (1)
An infant aged 1 month weighing 4 Kg requiring parenteral maintenance.
 Total fluid = $4 \times 150 = 600$ ml
 Total Calories = $4 \times 110 = 440$ Cals

Table 4.9 Infusion solutions providing Calories.

Infusion	Cals/L	Glucose gm/L	Fructose gm/L	Ethanol gm/L	Amino Acids gm/L	Nitrogen gm/L	Na mEq/L	K mEq/L
* Aminosol 10%	330	—	—	—	100	12·75	160	0·5
* Aminosol-Glucose	300	50	—	—	33	4·25	54	0·15
* Aminosol-Fructose-Ethanol	875	—	150	25	33	4·25	54	0·15
* Intralipid 20%	2000	—	—	—	—	—	—	—

* Manufactured by Vitrum, Sweden.

Maintenance sodium $= 4 \times 2 \cdot 5 = 10$ mEq
Maintenance potassium $= 4 \times 2 \cdot 5 = 10$ mEq
Of the Calories 70 per cent should ideally be as carbohydrate
i.e. $\dfrac{70}{100} \times \dfrac{440}{4} = 77$ gms

20 per cent of the energy should be provided by fat.
i.e. $\dfrac{20}{100} \times \dfrac{440}{9} = 10$ gms (approx) fat

10 per cent should be as protein
i.e. $\dfrac{10}{100} \times \dfrac{440}{4} = 11$ gm

200 ml of 'Aminosol-Fructose-Ethanol' would provide 10 mEq of sodium, an insignificant amount of potassium, about 5·1 gm of protein (0·85 gm of nitrogen) and 30 gm of fructose plus 5 gm of ethanol (together counted as 35 gm of carbohydrate).

The protein content is only about half the ideal, but more aminosol cannot be given as the sodium load would be too great.

Fat can be given as a total of 40 ml of 20 per cent 'Intralipid', i.e. 8 gms which is not far off requirements.

The remainder of the schedule must be constructed out of a dextrose or laevulose solution, and supplemental potassium chloride must also be given, some of which can be added to the 'Aminosol-Fructose-Ethanol' but *not* to the 'Intralipid'.

The schedule can therefore be written as a 24 hours requirement as shown in Table 4.10.

It will be noted that the schedule falls short of the optimum level of protein and carbohydrate intake, and the total Calories provided are barely sufficient. Herein lies the difficulty of maintaining the small infant by parenteral therapy in correct balance—with the infusions available one has to make a compromise with what is possible, bearing in mind the small volumes of fluid which can be used and the high sodium content of the 'Aminosol' solutions. However, the régime is an advance on what would be achieved by giving 600 ml of 5 per cent dextrose with saline, which would provide only 120 Cals without fat or protein.

Example (2)
A 4-year old child weighing 20 Kg, with high intestinal obstruction and continuous vomiting causing mild dehydration.

Table 4.10 4 Kg infant, 24 hours schedule of intravenous fluid.

Infusion solution	Volume	mEq Sodium	mEq Potassium	gm Protein	gm Fat	gm Carbohydrate	Calories
'Aminosol-Fructose-Ethanol'	200 ml +12·5 ml KCl (i.e.2½ ampoules)*	10	5	5·1	—	35	175
'Intra lipid' 20%	40 ml	—	—	—	8	—	80
10% Laevulose	335 ml +12·5 ml KCl*	—	5	—	—	33·5	134
TOTALS	600 ml	10	10	5·1	8·0	68·5	389

* 0.15 gm KCl to 5 ml.

Fluid, Electrolyte and Metabolic Balance 43

The biochemical findings might be: sodium 125 mEq/L, potassium 3·5 mEq/L, chloride 80 mEq/L and standard bicarbonate 35 mEq/L.

The vomiting has produced loss of water, hydrogen, sodium and chloride ions, causing a metabolic alkalosis. The fluid loss can be assessed as a 15 per cent deficit of extracellular fluid, and initial management is directed at a correction of the dehydration.

The extracellular compartment at this age would be 20 per cent of body weight, i.e. 4 litres. A 15 per cent deficit would amount to 600 ml and this should be made good by administration of 600 ml of normal saline in four hours, no attempt being made to give potassium, which would be dangerous in the presence of dehydration, or to correct the alkalotic state which will respond to improvement in renal function if the extracellular compartment is restored to normal. The total sodium deficit based on the formula:

$$(140-125) \times \text{total body water} = 15 \times \frac{65}{100} \times 20 = 195 \text{ mEq.}$$

600 ml of normal saline will provide only 92 mEq of sodium.

Following rehydration the biochemical findings might be: sodium 135 mEq/L, potassium 3·0 mEq/L, chloride 90 mEq/L, standard bicarbonate 30 mEq/L. The alkalosis is beginning to decrease.

The next twelve hours would involve the provision of a normal volume of fluid for age, and possibly more fluid to cope with the ongoing loss, if gastric aspiration were being employed. The sodium deficit must be made good and potassium should be given in slightly more than the maintenance level.

Total fluid/12 hours $= \frac{1}{2}$ of 24 hours volume
$\qquad = \frac{1}{2}$ of $20 \times 90 = 900$ ml

Sodium required/12 hours $= \frac{1}{2}$ of (maintenance+deficit)/24 hours
$\qquad \frac{1}{2}$ of $(2 \times 20) + (140-135) \times \frac{65}{100} \times 20$
$\qquad = 20 + 65$
$\qquad = 85$ mEq

Potassium required/12 hours $= \frac{1}{2}$ of (maintenance $+ \frac{1}{4}$ maintenance)/24 hours
$\qquad = \frac{1}{2}$ of $(40+10)$
$\qquad = 25$ mEq

The next 12 hours schedule would be shown in Table 4.11.

The following 24 hours would be concerned with the maintenance of normal fluid, electrolyte and Calorie balance, and the suggested

Table 4.11 20 Kg child, 12 hours repair schedule.

Infusion solution	Volume	Sodium mEq	Potassium mEq
Normal saline 500 ml + 13 mEq potassium chloride	Give 500 ml	77	13
5% dextrose 500 ml +13 mEq potassium chloride	Give 150 ml	—	3·9
0·18% sodium chloride 4·3% dextrose, 500 ml +13 mEq potassium chloride	Give 250 ml	7·7	6·5
TOTALS	900 ml	84·7	23·4

schedule would require modification if there were continuing losses e.g. gastric aspirate necessitating replacement therapy.

The ideal requirement would be:
Total fluid/24 hours = $20 \times 90 = 1,800$ ml
Total Calories/24 hours = $20 \times 80 = 1,600$ Cals
Sodium requirement/24 hours = 40 mEq
Potassium requirement/24 hours = 40 mEq
Protein = 40 gm
Carbohydrate = 280 gm
Fats = 35 gm

The suggested schedule would be as shown in Table 4.12.

Again within the electrolyte limitation imposed by the 'Aminosol' solution it has proved impossible to attain either the Calorie requirement or the theoretical optimum amount of protein and carbohydrate. The latter can only be supplied if one can afford to give *more* sodium than the maintenance dose, and therefore give a greater volume of 'Aminosol-Fructose-Ethanol'.

In most paediatric patients parenteral nutrition is required for only a relatively short time, and severe nitrogen depletion with profound wasting and hypoproteinaemic oedema is fortunately not often seen. The aim in treating any severely ill child is to resume alimentary feeding as soon as possible, owing to the inadequacies of parenteral therapy at the present time.

ADDENDUM

A recently introduced infusion solution ('Vamin', manufactured by

Table 4.12 Maintenance schedule for 24 hours. 20 Kg child.

Infusion solution	Volume	mEq Sodium	mEq Potassium	gm Protein	gm Fat	gm Carbohydrate	Calories
'Aminosol-Fructose-Ethanol' 1000 ml + 26 mEq KCl	Give 740 ml	40	20	19	—	129	642
'Intralipid' 20%	200 ml	—	—	—	40	—	400
10% Laevulose 1000 ml + 26 mEq KCl	Give 860 ml	—	22	—	—	43	172
TOTALS	1,800 ml	40	42	19	40	172	1,214

Vitrum of Stockholm) contains a greater proportion of nitrogen in relation to sodium than is the case with 'Aminosol-glucose' or 'Aminosol-Fructose-Ethanol'. The nitrogen is again provided as amino-acids in the laevo-form, and there is a significant amount of potassium. Each litre contains 9·4 gm of nitrogen, 50 mEq of sodium, 20 mEq of potassium, 5 mEq of Calcium, 3 mEq of magnesium, 55 mEq of chloride ion, together with 100 gm of fructose, and provides in all 650 Cals. Taking the basic amino-acid requirement as 1 gm/Kg of body weight and the example of the 20 Kg child given above it is still not possible to provide the theoretical nitrogen requirement, nor the required Calorie intake within the total fluid and sodium requirements. If both sodium and fluid can be increased above the theoretical total amount, then by giving 2 L of 'Vamin' plus 200 ml of 'Intralipid' an almost ideal infusion can be provided.

It has been reported that, in extremely ill children severe metabolic acidosis may follow infusion of fructose solutions if the rate exceeds 0·3gm/Kg/hour. The mechanism is unknown but high blood lactate levels are found. If unexpected tachypnoea and shock occur during parenteral nutrition, lactic acidosis must be considered as a possible explanation.

CHAPTER

5

Acid/Base Balance and Blood Gas Studies

In studying the effect of metabolic processes in the body it is important to have a readily available means of measuring the acidity or alkalinity of the blood. Chemical indicators (such as litmus) cannot be employed owing to the small magnitude of the changes involved.

pH is a means of measurement of the acidity or alkalinity of a solution, that is, it is a measurement of the hydrogen ion concentration. By definition, an acid is a substance which dissociates in aqueous solution to form a hydrogen ion and a negative ion (anion). For example, hydrochloric acid:

$HCl \rightleftharpoons H^+ + Cl^-$

A base is a substance which will accept hydrogen ions.

The degree of acidity of a solution can therefore be measured by recording the concentration of hydrogen ions, but when expressed in terms of g/litre this number is very small. (Table 5.1). It is more

Table 5.1 Relationship between hydrogen ion concentration and pH.

$[H^+]$	pH
0·000,000,158	6·82
0·000,000,040	7·40
0·000,000,015	7·82

convenient to express hydrogen ion concentration in the form of pH, which is the negative logarithm of the hydrogen ion concentration.

$pH = -\log [H^+]$

This brings the expression of hydrogen ion concentration into the form of a whole number; the range extends from 0–14, a neutral solution having a pH of 7·00. Blood has a pH range of 7·36 to 7·44, and small deviations from this can cause symptoms. An *increase* in pH reflects a *decrease* in the hydrogen ion concentration, and vice versa.

Acidosis may be defined as the condition in which arterial pH is below the normal range, while in *alkalosis* the pH is greater than normal. Respiratory acid/base disturbances are due to alveolar hypoventilation or hyperventilation, leading respectively to accumulation or to washing out of carbon dioxide. Metabolic disturbances result in an accumulation or loss of acid or base from sources other than carbon dioxide.

The partial pressure of a gas is another concept which requires explanation. In a mixture of gases the pressure exerted by one gas is called its partial pressure, and the sum of the partial pressures gives the pressure of the gas mixture as a whole. Thus the sum of the partial pressures of the various gases present in air, plus the pressure exerted by water vapour, is equal to the atmospheric pressure. $P_{A}co_2$ is the symbol used to describe the partial pressure of carbon dioxide in alveolar gas, and $P_{a}co_2$ the partial pressure in arterial blood; at a temperature of 38°C and with the haemoglobin fully saturated with oxygen these are normally both 40 mm mercury (40 mm Hg). A $P_{a}co_2$ of higher than normal indicates failure to eliminate carbon dioxide properly (*respiratory acidosis*) and will cause a lowering of pH. *Respiratory alkalosis* is said to exist when the $P_{a}co_2$ is below normal and the pH will rise. Compensatory mechanisms usually come into operation to limit the rise or fall of pH.

Compensation for changes in hydrogen ion concentration is effected by the *buffer systems*, which are designed to maintain pH at or near to normal. The capacity of a buffer is expressed as the rate of change of pH when acid or base is added. A buffer, chemically speaking, is a partially ionized salt formed by the combination of a strong acid and a weak base, or vice versa. A buffer system usually consists of a *pair* of substances, and is most effective when both the salt and the weak acid or base are present in equal quantities. Thus a *buffer pair* can be represented as follows:

$$HA \rightleftharpoons H^+ + A^- \quad (1)$$
$$BA \rightleftharpoons B^+ + A^- \quad (2)$$

Acid/Base Balance and Blood Gas Studies

Addition of hydrogen ions to this system would cause the chemical equilibrium in equation (1) to move to the left, that is, more of the acid would be present in the non-dissociated form. The resultant decrease of anions is compensated by further dissociation of the salt, so that the chemical equilibrium in equation (2) moves to the right. The converse will happen if base is added to the buffer mixture.

In the blood there are four buffer systems concerned in the defences of the body against pH variations. They are:

(i) The haemoglobin–oxyhaemoglobin system. The buffering capacity of haemoglobin depends on the fact that oxyhaemoglobin is a stronger acid than reduced haemoglobin. At a given pH, therefore, more base must be combined with oxyhaemoglobin than with reduced haemoglobin. In the lungs this can be represented as follows:

$H.Hb + O_2 \longrightarrow H.HbO_2$ where $H.Hb$ is acid reduced haemoglobin and $H.HbO_2$ is acid oxyhaemoglobin.

$H.HbO_2 + BHCO_3 \longrightarrow B.HbO_2 + H_2CO_3$

$H_2CO_3 \longrightarrow H_2O + CO_2$ in expired air

In the tissues oxygen is released and reduced haemoglobin is formed combined with base as buffered reduced haemoglobin.

$B.HbO_2 \longrightarrow B.Hb + O_2$ Where $B.HbO_2$ is buffered oxyhaemoglobin and $B.Hb$ is buffered reduced haemoglobin.

Tissue metabolism results in the liberation of carbon dioxide which combines with water to form carbonic acid in the red cell under the influence of carbonic anhydrase.

$$CO_2 + H_2O \xrightarrow{\text{carbonic anhydrase}} H_2CO_3$$

This then reacts with the buffered reduced haemoglobin to form acid reduced haemoglobin and base.

$H_2CO_3 + B.Hb \longrightarrow H.Hb + B.HCO_3$

The cycle then repeats when the acid reduced haemoglobin reaches the lungs.

This buffering action of haemoglobin accounts for the supply of sufficient base for the transport of over half the carbon dioxide in the blood.

(ii) The blood proteins. These have the ability to act as either acids or bases, and therefore each protein acts as a buffer pair.

(iii) The phosphates. Na_2HPO_4/NaH_2PO_4

(iv) The bicarbonate-carbon dioxide system. This may be explained by considering the equation:

$$CO_2 + H_2O \rightleftharpoons H_2CO_3 \rightleftharpoons H^+ + HCO_3^-$$

If hydrogen ions are added the system will shift to the left, as some of the hydrogen ions combine with bicarbonate ions. Alternatively if hydrogen ions are removed by adding base, further dissociation of carbonic acid occurs to form more hydrogen ions.

The buffer pair in this system is $NaHCO_3/H_2CO_3$, and this buffer system is the one most commonly used to assess acid/base balance. Its immediate readiness for action in the body is determined by the availability of bicarbonate ion, and by the efficacy of elimination of carbon dioxide by the lungs.

The efficiency of the blood buffers can be illustrated simply. If a drop of very dilute hydrochloric acid is added to 100 ml of distilled water at pH 7·35, the pH would fall to 7·00. With 100 ml of blood about 25 *ml* of acid would be needed to achieve the same pH change.

In evaluating the acid/base state of a patient, repeated measurements may be needed, and this has been greatly assisted by microbiochemical methods using the Astrup technique. The pH, P_aco_2 and standard bicarbonate* are estimated and are mutually dependent on one another according to the Henderson-Hasselbalch equation:

$$pH = pK + \log \frac{HCO_3^-}{H_2CO_3}$$ where pK is a dissociation constant

or alternatively:

$$pH = pK + \log \frac{HCO_3^-}{S \times P_aco_2}$$

where S is the solubility of carbon dioxide in the plasma.

Bicarbonate is controlled by metabolic processes in the body producing it, and by renal excretion, that is, non-respiratory mechanisms, whilst P_aco_2 is controlled by respiratory mechanisms.

Most metabolic processes in the body liberate hydrogen ions. The cellular metabolism of glucose progresses to lactate, later converted to bicarbonate, while fatty acids liberate acetic acid. Normally, further oxidation proceeds to carbon dioxide (eliminated by the

* The standard bicarbonate is a measurement of bicarbonate in fully oxygenated blood at a temperature of 38°C and with a partial pressure of carbon dioxide of 40 mm Hg.

lungs) and water. *Anaerobic* metabolism of glucose leads to the accumulation of lactic and pyruvic acids, requiring buffering by the blood and utilization of bicarbonate. Deranged fat metabolism, as in diabetes mellitus, will also result in metabolic acidosis. In normal individuals, during severe exercise, a transient excess of acid metabolites occurs with a slight fall of pH, but the blood buffers will cope with the excess acid, and increased ventilation eliminates as much carbon dioxide as possible. Excess hydrogen ions are also removed in part by renal excretion, although this is a much slower mechanism.

Most of the carbon dioxide in the blood is carried in the red cells. After diffusion through the red cell wall, under the influence of the enzyme carbonic anhydrase, carbonic acid is produced. Some of this returns to the plasma, but the remainder is buffered inside the red cell by potassium in association with reduced haemoglobin. This chemical reaction results in the production of potassium bicarbonate.

$$H_2CO_3 + K.Hb \longrightarrow H.Hb + KHCO_3$$

The red cell wall is impermeable to sodium and potassium ions, but permeable to hydrogen, bicarbonate and chloride ions. Chloride from the plasma is thought to exchange with bicarbonate in the red cell, forming sodium bicarbonate in the plasma and potassium chloride in the red cell.

This can be represented diagramatically (Fig. 5.1)

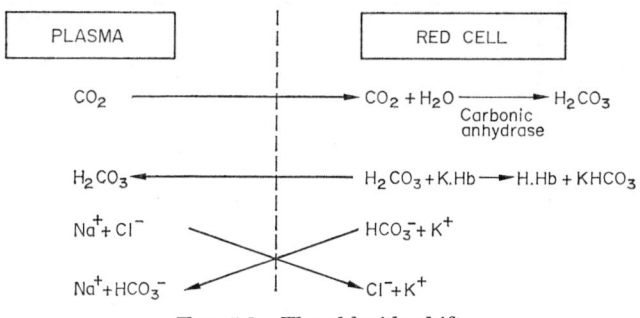

FIG. 5.1 The chloride shift.

This movement of chloride from the plasma into the red cells is called the *chloride shift*, and has a practical importance in the consideration of the acid/base state which will be discussed later.

The interrelationship of pH, P_aco_2 and bicarbonate can be represented diagramatically in the form of a balance (Fig. 5.2).

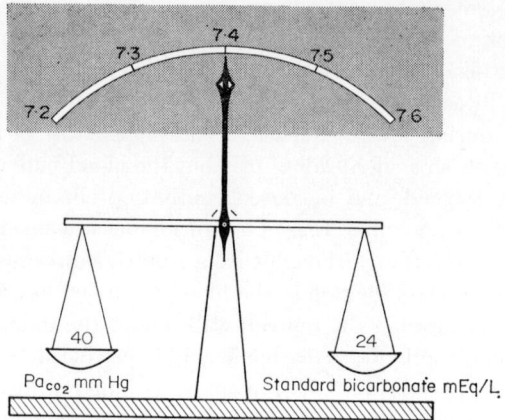

Fig. 5.2 P_aCO_2/Bicarbonate Balance.

A change in one side of the balance, unless accompanied by a change on the other, will be revealed as a change in pH. Usually the change is modified by compensatory mechanisms to maintain the pH as near normal as possible. The possible acid/base disturbances are shown (Table 5.2).

Table 5.2 Common acid/base disturbances.

Acid/base Disturbances	pH	P_aCO_2	Standard Bicarbonate
Respiratory acidosis e.g. Acute Respiratory Failure	Lowered	Raised	Normal or raised
Respiratory Alkalosis e.g. Hyperventilation	Raised	Lowered	Normal or lowered
Non-respiratory Acidosis e.g. Acute Renal Failure	Lowered	Lowered	Lowered
Non-respiratory Alkalosis e.g. vomiting	Raised	Raised	Raised

In respiratory acidosis the rise of bicarbonate necessary to compensate for the high P_aCO_2 is achieved by the kidney retaining bicarbonate ion and excreting hydrogen ion.

In hyperventilation, the reverse change occurs, the kidney retaining hydrogen ion and excreting bicarbonate.

A patient who has a high standard bicarbonate (i.e. high pH) will

Acid/Base Balance and Blood Gas Studies

often hypoventilate, the effect of this being to raise the $P_a\text{CO}_2$ and lower the pH.

A patient who has a low standard bicarbonate (low pH) often compensates by hyperventilation, which lowers the $P_a\text{CO}_2$ and raises the pH.

In general, compensatory mechanisms for low pH are more efficient than those for high pH, and there is a limit in any case to the degree of compensation which the body can achieve.

Measurements in Assessing Acid/Base Disturbances

It is essential to employ arterial blood for accurate determination of pH and $P\text{CO}_2$. The blood is taken into a heparinized syringe (about 5 ml) and the syringe is then sealed with a cap. If there is likely to be any delay in analysis the syringe is kept on ice. In paediatric practice, however, particularly when dealing with infants, repeated arterial punctures are difficult and probably undesirable in view of the danger of repeated trauma to tiny vessels. *Provided* that the peripheral circulation is *good* without stasis, and provided that the capillary blood can be obtained easily by cutaneous puncture without undue pressure, capillary samples give valid results. It may be necessary to provide local warmth to the part before making the puncture.

The technical details of the estimations are not important in the present context, but if required can be obtained from standard reference works. The micro-technique devised by Astrup is employed, and all measurements are carried out at 38°C. (If the patient's temperature is significantly lower than this a correction of the results must be made.)

The pH is measured using a glass electrode. The carbon dioxide tension is measured by the technique developed by Severinghaus, in which the glass electrode is surrounded by a bicarbonate buffer and separated from the blood sample by a plastic gas-permeable membrane. Calibration is achieved by using water or saline, equilibrated with different carbon dioxide concentrations. The sample is then measured with the electrode; carbon dioxide diffuses through the membrane into the bicarbonate solution, causing a change in pH that is recorded by the glass electrode.

The Astrup technique measures the pH and the $P_a\text{CO}_2$. After recording the pH of the sample it is then exposed to two gas mixtures of known $P\text{CO}_2$ values, and the pH is measured at each of these. Suitable gas mixtures of oxygen and carbon dioxide employed would give a $P\text{CO}_2$ of approximately 30 and 65 mm Hg (correction for barometric pressure is necessary; e.g. carbon dioxide 4 per cent, oxygen 96 per cent in cylinder, atmospheric pressure 750 mm Hg, $P\text{CO}_2 = \frac{4}{100} \times 750 = 30$ mm Hg; using the same gas mixture but atmospheric pressure 755 mm Hg, $P\text{CO}_2 = \frac{4}{100} \times 755 = 30 \cdot 2$ mm Hg). This gives two co-ordinates of pH and $P\text{CO}_2$ which can be plotted on a suitable graph such as the Siggaard-Andersen curve nomogram (Fig. 5.3).

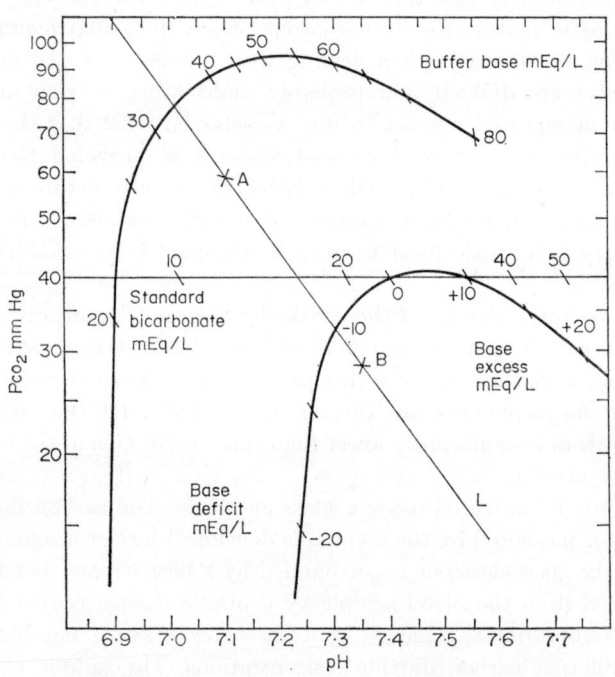

FIG. 5.3 Siggaard-Andersen nomogram (modified).

By drawing a line through the two co-ordinates it will be found to cut the buffer base curve, the base excess/deficit curve, and the

Acid/Base Balance and Blood Gas Studies

standard bicarbonate line, and the appropriate values of these can be read off.

For example, if the pH at $P\text{co}_2$ 60 mm Hg is 7·1, and at 30 mm Hg it is 7·34, these two points A and B are plotted on the graph. The line between them, L, cuts the buffer base curve at 33 mEq/L, the standard bicarbonate line at 17 mEq/L and the base deficit curve at −10 mEq/L.

Note that on the graph at a $P\text{co}_2$ of 40 mm Hg, and a pH of 7·4, the base excess is zero.

In addition to the above the sample is used to measure the serum sodium, potassium and chloride. This gives a useful check on the laboratory estimation of standard bicarbonate, and depends on the interrelationship of chloride and bicarbonate ion (q.v. the chloride shift). Normally, unless there are excesses of other serum anions the serum sodium should be related to bicarbonate and chloride according to the equation.

Serum Na mEq/L=standard bicarbonate mEq/L+serum chloride mEq/L+10.
e.g. Serum Na = 24+105+10
= 139 mEq/L.

The Determination and Use of P_aO_2

Just as $P_a\text{co}_2$ is the measurement of the partial pressure exerted by carbon dioxide in arterial blood, so P_aO_2 is the partial pressure exerted by oxygen, and this depends on oxygen diffusing across the alveolar membrane without any hindrance, and on the partial pressure of oxygen in alveolar gas (P_AO_2).

At standard barometric pressure of 760 mm Hg the partial pressure of oxygen in air would be approximately one fifth of this (oxygen being 20·9 per cent of air), that is 159 mm Hg. The Po_2 can always be calculated in a gas mixture providing the fraction of the *dry* gas present as oxygen is known (this fraction is represented as F).

Thus $Po_2 = Fo_2 \times PB$

where PB is the barometric pressure.

If the gas mixture is saturated with water vapour then the partial pressure of water vapour (47 mm Hg) has to be subtracted from the barometric pressure.

Then $Po_2 = Fo_2 (PB - 47)$

If we consider inspired gas (e.g. an anaesthetic mixture)
$PIo_2 = FIo_2 (PB - 47)$
Since the partial pressure of oxygen in inspired gas 'drives' oxygen across the alveolar membrane into the blood the partial pressures on both sides of the membrane are very similar; e.g. P_{AO_2} 100 mm Hg, P_aO_2 95 mm Hg.

The difference between the two oxygen tensions is called the A—a gradient, in the above instance being 5 mm Hg.

It will be noted that the PIo_2 of air would be about 149 mm Hg $\left(\text{calculated as } \frac{20 \cdot 9}{100} \times (760-47)\right)$ and that this is considerably higher than the P_{AO_2}.

The reason for the difference is the fact that some oxygen has diffused from alveolar gas into the blood, and an equilibrium has been reached.

P_aO_2 is measured in a sample of heparinized arterial blood collected as already described, care being taken to avoid introducing air into the syringe. A Clark electrode is employed; this is made of platinum, surrounded by electrolyte, and separated from the blood sample by a plastic, gas-permeable membrane. The electrode measures the breakdown of oxygen molecules, at the platinum surface after they have diffused from the blood into the electrolyte. Calibration is achieved by reading the pH on a pH meter, using samples of water exposed to varying known oxygen tensions. The P_aO_2 is then measured, the temperature being 38°C: if the patient's temperature is below this a correction must be carried out.

It is useful to check the laboratory measurement of P_aO_2 by working out the approximate P_{AO_2}. Supposing a patient is receiving a mixture of 50 per cent oxygen and 50 per cent air. The FIo_2 would be 50 per cent $+1/5$ 50 per cent $= 60$ per cent

$P_{AO_2} \simeq FIo_2 (PB - P_aCO_2 - P_{H_2O})$.

Where PB = barometric pressure, P_aCO_2 is measured for the individual patient, and P_{H_2O} is the partial pressure of water vapour.

Supposing in this particular instance P_aCO_2 is 40 mm Hg.
$P_{AO_2} \simeq \frac{60}{100} (760 - 40 - 47)$
$\simeq \frac{3}{5} \times 673$
$\simeq 404$ mm Hg

Since the P_aO_2 cannot be *more* than the P_{AO_2} and indeed is always less, this gives a useful rough check against technical errors in the laboratory.

If the measured $P_{a O_2}$ is considerably less than the estimated $P_{A O_2}$ it would suggest that the A—a gradient is greater than normal and by implication that there is some difficulty in diffusion of oxygen across the alveolar membrane, or that a shunt is operating within the lung whereby desaturated blood bypasses the alveolar capillaries to reach the pulmonary veins without picking up oxygen.

The Correction of Acid/Base Disturbances and Disordered Blood Gas Tensions

It cannot be over emphasized that correction of disturbances of acid/base balance and the blood gases must be directed to treatment of the *cause* of the *deranged physiology*. To take an example, the ketoacidosis of diabetic coma causing a severe lowering of pH can be treated as an emergency measure by intravenous administration of sodium bicarbonate solution, and this may be life-saving. However, the cause of the coma, disordered fat metabolism secondary to faulty carbohydrate metabolism, requires the appropriate measures.

Again, whenever there is a low cardiac output with tissue hypoxia and a poor peripheral circulation, a metabolic acidosis will occur due to the accumulation of acid metabolites (lactic and pyruvic acids) with depletion of bicarbonate. To give intravenous bicarbonate to restore the pH to normal will produce only temporary improvement, and measures must be taken to improve tissue perfusion.

In most instances of severe bicarbonate depletion it is advisable to administer bicarbonate in addition to giving the other appropriate treatment. A useful formula to calculate the amount required is:

Sodium bicarbonate mEq = base deficit mEq/L × body weight in Kg × 0·3.

The formula is based on correcting the deficit in the extracellular fluid (taken to be 30 per cent of body weight) and this is therefore an *undercorrection*. However, if *very large* quantities of bicarbonate are given intravenously, a severe alkalosis can result which is slow to resolve.

Two examples may serve to illustrate the use made of the acid/base and blood gas data:

(a) *Acute on Chronic Respiratory Failure:* for example, a child with bronchopneumonia superimposed on severe fibrocystic disease of the lungs. The data obtained might be: pH 7·14; P_aco_2 120 mm Hg; standard bicarbonate 25·5 mEq/L; base excess+1·5 mEq/L; P_aO_2 30 mm Hg.

These results show that the child has a severe uncompensated respiratory acidosis with severe hypoxia. The reasons why compensation by means of a raised standard bicarbonate is not occurring are:

(i) The infection is causing protein breakdown, with the liberation of hydrogen ions, thus using up bicarbonate.

(ii) Hypoxia leads to anaerobic metabolism of carbohydrate with accumulation of acid metabolites, which also removes bicarbonate.

(iii) Hypoxia and circulatory failure will tend to produce renal shutdown so that the kidney cannot excrete excess hydrogen ions.

Treatment must be directed towards two main aims, that is to the control of infection, and to the improvement of pulmonary ventilation so ensuring adequate elimination of carbon dioxide and the raising of P_aO_2. The second of these may necessitate artificial ventilation of the lungs.

(b) *Acute renal failure:* this is accompanied by a low urine output with a low urea concentration, and a rising serum urea and potassium. Hydrogen ions cannot be excreted, so the standard bicarbonate falls. Hyperventilation may compensate for this by lowering the Pco_2. The data obtained might be:

pH 7·33; P_aco_2 24 mm Hg; standard bicarbonate 15·5 mEq/L; base deficit—11·5 mEq/L.

Such a patient may require dialysis if the serum urea and potassium continue to rise, the aim being to remove urea, potassium and hydrogen ions, and to replace bicarbonate. It is often found that after dialysis, although the pH and standard bicarbonate have been restored to normal, the patient may continue to hyperventilate. The reason for this is that the *intracellular* pH is still low. One must always remember that acid/base measurements are made on extracellular fluid, and do not necessarily reflect the intracellular state.

Terms Used and Normal Values

Pco_2 —the partial pressure of carbon dioxide in mm Hg.
P_Aco_2 —the partial pressure of carbon dioxide in alveolar gas. Normal 40 mm Hg.

P_aCO_2 —the partial pressure of carbon dioxide in arterial blood. Normal 40 mm Hg.
PO_2 —the partial pressure of oxygen in mm Hg.
PIO_2 —the partial pressure of oxygen in inspired gas.
P_AO_2 —the partial pressure of oxygen in alveolar gas. Normal 100 mm Hg.
P_aO_2 —the partial pressure of oxygen in arterial blood. Normal 95 mm Hg.
F —the fraction of dry gas in a gas mixture.
FIO_2 —the fraction of oxygen in inspired gas.
pH —the negative logarithm of the hydrogen ion concentration. Normal range for blood 7·36 to 7·44.
Standard bicarbonate —the bicarbonate in fully oxygenated blood at a temperature of 38°C and with a PCO_2 of 40 mm Hg. Normal range for blood 22–26 mEq/L.

FURTHER READING

DAVENPORT, H. W. (1969) *The ABC of Acid-Base Chemistry*, University of Chicago Press.

SIGGAARD-ANDERSEN O. (1946) *The Acid-Base Status of the Blood*, Williams & Wilkins Co.

CHAPTER 6

Respiratory Physiology

The function of the lungs is to oxygenate venous blood and to eliminate excess carbon dioxide from it. These aims are accomplished by diffusion of the gases between the blood and the alveoli, across the alveolar walls. As air enters the alveoli, gas diffusion takes place until the mixture has a uniform composition in which there is only a small alteration during the respiratory cycle. Alveolar gas contains 14 volumes per cent of oxygen, 5·6 volumes per cent of carbon dioxide and the rest is water vapour and nitrogen. Gases always diffuse in the direction of lower partial pressure, but the pressure is not necessarily an indication of concentration, because of the solubility of the gas in water—a relatively insoluble gas, e.g. oxygen, will exert a high partial pressure at a low concentration, but a very soluble gas, such as carbon dioxide, must reach a high dissolved concentration before it will exert the same partial pressure. Therefore, it is better to speak in terms of pressure than concentration. The partial pressures of gases in various parts of the respiratory cycle are as in Table 6.1.

Table 6.1 Partial pressures of gases in respiratory cycle mm Hg

	P_{O_2}	P_{CO_2}	P_{N_2}	P_{H_2O}
atmosphere	159	0·3	601	0
inspired gas	149	0·3	564	47
expired gas	116	28	569	47
alveolar gas	100	40	573	47
arterial gas	95	40	573	47
venous blood	40	46	573	47

Respiratory Physiology

From this it can be seen that the pressure gradient from alveolus to blood for oxygen is 100 mm Hg to 40 mm Hg, and that for carbon dioxide from blood to alveolus is 46 mm Hg to 40 mm Hg. As carbon dioxide is so soluble this small pressure gradient is sufficient for the release of large volumes of gas.

The pulmonary vasculature consists of arteries and arterioles, carrying poorly oxygenated blood; capillaries, which are situated in the walls of the alveoli; and venules and veins, carrying oxygenated blood to the heart.

The whole of the cardiac output must pass through the lungs but the actual volume of blood in the pulmonary capillaries at any time is quite small—75 to 100 ml in the resting adult. Ideally it should be evenly distributed throughout both lungs, but in fact there is always some unevenness of distribution, one cause being gravity—most marked in the upright position, when there is more blood in the lung bases than in the apices.

If cardiac output falls severely, as in shock, some of the vascular channels close. In exercise, when the increased muscular metabolism demands large supplies of oxygenated blood, the blood flow through the lungs is greatly increased and more capillaries may open up to accommodate the load. This can normally be accomplished without much rise in pulmonary artery pressure, provided the lungs and blood vessels are healthy.

The pulmonary circulation will be more fully discussed in Chapter 7.

CONTROL OF VENTILATION

Ventilation, or the rhythmical expansion and deflation of the lungs and thorax, is an automatic process, and is controlled by aggregations of nervous tissue in the brain stem, collectively called the respiratory centre (R.C.). This centre is influenced by the pneumotaxic centre in the midbrain, and by the cerebral cortex.

The activity of the R.C. is also influenced by information from several other sources. The vagus nerves carry information about the state of inflation of the lungs; sensory nerves carry proprioceptive impulses from skeletal muscles and joints; specialised nervous tissue in the carotid and aortic bodies is chemoreceptor and affected by the oxygenation and acid/base state of the blood. Hypoxia and metabolic acidosis cause stimulation of the R.C. through these bodies. However, the most sensitive control of the R.C. is exerted by the arterial $P\text{CO}_2$, which has a direct action on the centre. An increase in $P_a\text{CO}_2$ stimulates respiration, normally by an increase in tidal volume rather than rate. The centre is eventually depressed by both hypercarbia and hypoxia.

Impulses from the R.C. are carried by motor nerves to the muscles of respiration.

MECHANICS OF VENTILATION

On inspiration, contraction of the intercostal muscles causes the lower ribs to move upwards and outwards, thereby increasing both transverse and antero-posterior dimensions of the thorax. The volume of the thoracic cage is further increased by downward movement of the diaphragm. Both the internal surface of the thoracic cage and the external surface of the lung are covered by a thin layer of cells forming the pleurae—parietal and visceral respectively—and between the layers is a film of fluid. The surface tension properties of this fluid keep the two surfaces together, so that the lung follows the movements of the chest wall. The lung is an elastic structure which resists expansion, but it is forced to do so as the chest wall expands and a negative pressure is created between the layers of pleura. This pressure can be measured by a balloon placed in the oesophagus. As the lung expands, air flows through the open larynx until the pressure nears atmospheric. There is resistance to air flow in the airways and, to overcome this, as well as the elasticity of the lung, muscular work must be done. If the lungs or airways are abnormal, extra work is required, and accessory muscles of inspiration, such as the sternomastoids and scaleni, are used. Intercostal recession may also be present, especially in babies.

When the expanding force stops working, and the muscles relax at the end of inspiration, the lungs deflate due to their elastic properties, driving air out, and causing the chest wall to return to its original position. In normal expiration muscular effort is not required, and the expiratory muscles are used only in coughing and straining, or if there is resistance to expiration, as in asthma.

Deflation of the lung is assisted by the surface tension properties of a special fluid, surfactant, lining the alveoli. It is a lipoprotein, and its surface tension is variable, according to the state of inflation of the lungs—greatest when they are expanded, and decreasing as they deflate, so that the alveoli never close completely. If this fluid had ordinary properties, surface tension would increase as the size of the alveoli decreased, and this would cause alveolar collapse, requiring a large force to re-expand them for the next inspiration. This happens with the first breath taken after birth, and also in the condition of respiratory distress syndrome of the newborn, which is thought to be caused by a lack of surfactant.

Compliance is a term used to describe the elastic properties of the lung and thorax. It is defined as the increase in lung volume per unit increase in distending pressure. The units are litres/cmH_2O. If only a small increase in volume is produced by a high distending pressure, the compliance is low, and the lungs feel 'stiff', and vice versa. If compliance is to be compared in different patients it must be related to the functional residual capacity of the lung. This is called the specific compliance, which is similar at all age groups, provided the lungs are normal.

Resistance is the pressure differential required to produce a unit flow change along a tube and the units are cm H_2O/litres/sec. It refers to the resistance offered by the airways to the passage of air along them. If resistance is high, there must be a large pressure difference between the mouth and the alveoli, for air flow to occur. Resistance to flow is proportional to the length of the tube, and inversely proportional to the fourth power of the radius of that tube (Poiseuille's law). This is obviously important in paediatrics.

The *time constant* of the lung is found by multiplying compliance and resistance.

L/cmH_2O × cmH_2O/L/sec = time in seconds.

It is the time taken for 63 per cent completion of expiration. After the passage of five time constants, the process of expiration is 99 per cent complete. This measurement is relevant in asthma, because prolonged expiration is required when airway resistance is high. In artificial ventilation it is useful to have some idea of the time constant, as it is pointless to prolong inspiration after three time constants have elapsed. Experiments have shown that a very short inspiratory time gives maldistribution of gas.

LUNG VOLUMES

The volume of gas taken into the lungs during a normal quiet inspiration is called the *tidal volume* (T.V.), and its magnitude is governed largely by tissue production of carbon dioxide.

Minute volume (M.V.) is T.V. ×rate. The rate of ventilation is governed by the R.C. and will increase if the work of breathing increases. Infants have a high resting rate of ventilation.

At the end of quiet expiration, the volume of gas left in the lungs is called the *functional residual capacity* (F.R.C.). It is increased in emphysema.

At the end of a forced expiration, the volume left is the *residual volume* (R.V.).

Vital capacity (V.C.) is the volume of air expelled by a maximum voluntary expiration after a maximum voluntary inspiration. It is a useful measure of pulmonary function in co-operative patients. The $F.E.V._1$ is another measurement used. It is the proportion of the forced vital capacity expelled after one second. These measurements are traced on paper by a spirograph, and from the shape of the curve the time constant and the type of lung disease can be deduced.

ALVEOLAR VENTILATION AND DEAD SPACE

Of the resting tidal volume, about one-third merely fills the airways and does not take part in gas exchange. This volume is called the *anatomical dead space*, and is said to be roughly equal to the body weight in pounds.

The remainder of the tidal volume enters the alveoli, mixes with gas already present, and takes part in gas exchange with the blood. This is termed *alveolar ventilation*.

Since the volume of the airways is constant for a particular subject, a decrease in tidal volume will mean a decrease in alveolar ventilation, and there will be interference with gas exchange. To achieve adequate elimination of carbon dioxide the tidal volume will have to be increased. If disease makes this impossible, then the rate must increase, or P_aco_2 will rise.

Ideally, the distribution of gas and blood throughout the lung should be even, and it is the relationship between the two which ensures normal blood gas values.

In the adult $\dfrac{\text{alveolar ventilation}}{\text{cardiac output}} = \dfrac{4 \text{ L/min}}{5 \text{ L/min}} = 0\cdot 8$

Respiratory Physiology

This is the *respiratory exchange ratio*, and should be the same for all alveoli.

In fact the ideal is never achieved for all alveoli. Some are ventilated but have no blood flowing through them and others are ventilated excessively for the amount of blood flow. These parts of the alveolar ventilation are wasted as far as gas exchange goes, and are called *alveolar dead space ventilation*. This volume, plus the anatomical dead space, make up the *physiological dead space*.

On the other hand, some alveoli may have blood supply but no ventilation, or insufficient ventilation. In this case, some blood enters the pulmonary veins incompletely oxygenated—a venous admixture effect, or *shunt*, and some degree of arterial haemoglobin desaturation will occur if the patient is breathing air.

Although overventilated alveoli will eliminate more carbon dioxide and compensate for its retention in underventilated alveoli, inequality of oxygen uptake cannot be fully compensated for in this way. Overventilation causes little increase in oxygen taken up by the blood, because of the shape of the haemoglobin dissociation curve. If total ventilation is increased, to improve ventilation in underventilated alveoli, and so improve oxygenation, the P_aco_2 will be lowered. Local adjustments tend to take place in the lungs to keep the ventilation : perfusion ratios normal—for instance, if ventilation to one lung is stopped, the pulmonary artery to this lung will constrict. The mechanism for this is not known.

DIFFUSION

Gas diffusion across the alveolar walls is an essential part of respiration, and is affected by many factors. However, pure disorders of diffusion are seldom severe enough to cause anoxaemia at rest. Carbon dioxide diffuses twenty times more rapidly than oxygen, and diffusion disorders are never a cause of carbon dioxide retention.

The distance across which diffusion must occur consists of the alveolar fluid, alveolar membrane, capillary membrane, plasma, and red blood cell membrane, and an increase in thickness of any of these layers will retard diffusion. The rate of uptake of oxygen by the haemoglobin is also a factor.

The diffusing capacity for oxygen is difficult to measure, and that for carbon monoxide is usually measured instead. Carbon monoxide has a high affinity for haemoglobin, and is taken up in preference to oxygen. This is why carbon monoxide poisoning leads to hypoxia.

BLOOD GAS TRANSPORT

Oxygen

A small amount of oxygen is carried in solution in the plasma, and this is important, because it determines the P_aO_2. This volume, in a normal patient breathing air, is 0·3 vols per cent. The great bulk of the oxygen carried in the blood is present in chemical combination with haemoglobin inside the red blood cells. The combination is a loose one, and easily broken when oxygen must be released to the tissues.

At a tension of 100 mm Hg or more, the haemoglobin is fully saturated with oxygen. Then 1·34 ml O_2 are combined with each gramme of haemoglobin. The actual volume carried depends on Po_2 and on the haemoglobin concentration. The arterial blood oxygen saturation is often measured—this relates the actual amount of oxygen present to the capacity of the blood for holding oxygen.

$$\text{per cent saturation} = \frac{\text{ml } O_2 \text{ actually combined with Hb}}{O_2 \text{ carrying capacity of Hb}}$$

The relationship between partial pressure of oxygen in the blood and the per cent saturation is expressed in the haemoglobin dissociation curve for oxygen.

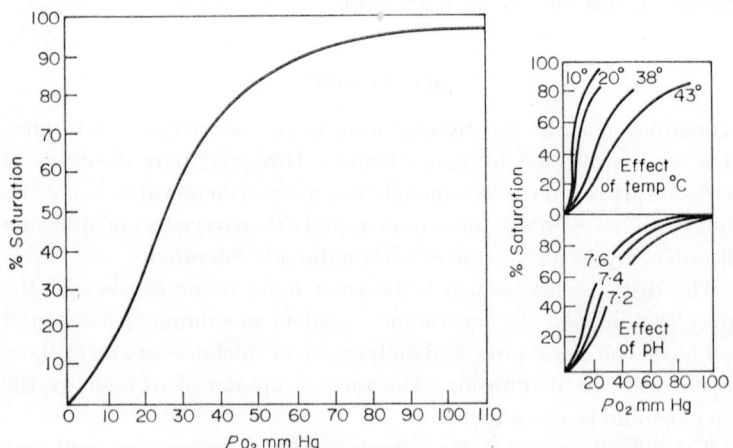

FIG. 6.1 Oxygen dissociation curve.

Respiratory Physiology

The fact that the curve is S shaped holds great advantages for the body, because, even though the P_aO_2 may fall to 80 mm Hg the haemoglobin will still be almost fully saturated. An increase in P_aO_2 above 100 mm Hg causes very little extra uptake of oxygen. The steep part of the curve signifies that a drop of P_aO_2 below 60 mm Hg causes a large volume of oxygen to be released from the haemoglobin, and this occurs in the tissues, assisted by movement of carbon dioxide in the reverse direction. A P_aO_2 below 30 mm Hg for any length of time is incompatible with life.

The slope of the curve is affected by factors such as a rise in blood P_{CO_2}, increased hydrogen ion concentration, and raised temperature, all of which shift the curve across to the right, thereby facilitating the release of oxygen to the tissues. The reverse conditions shift the curve to the left.

Carbon dioxide

Carbon dioxide is produced by cellular metabolism in the tissues, enters the blood, and is carried in three forms—in simple solution (8 per cent), as bicarbonate (65 per cent) and in chemical combination with proteins, chiefly haemoglobin, as carbamino-haemoglobin (27 per cent).

Carbon dioxide in simple solution in the plasma slowly forms carbonic acid, but this reaction is very much faster in the red cells, facilitated by the enzyme carbonic anhydrase. Carbon dioxide diffuses from the tissues into the plasma, and into the red cells, there to be converted to carbonic acid, which dissociates into bicarbonate ions.

$$H_2CO_3 \rightleftharpoons H^+ + HCO_3$$

The bicarbonate ions diffuse out into the plasma, and chloride ions diffuse in, to maintain electrical neutrality.

Some of the carbon dioxide in the red cell enters into chemical combination with haemoglobin and this assists the release of oxygen to the tissues. The reverse reactions occur in the lungs. It can be seen that red cells are important in carbon dioxide transport.

Just as with oxygen, the relationship between P_aCO_2 and total CO_2 content can be expressed as a dissociation curve.

Note that this curve is almost linear, so an increase or decrease in P_aCO_2 can be compensated for in the lungs. The curve is steep,

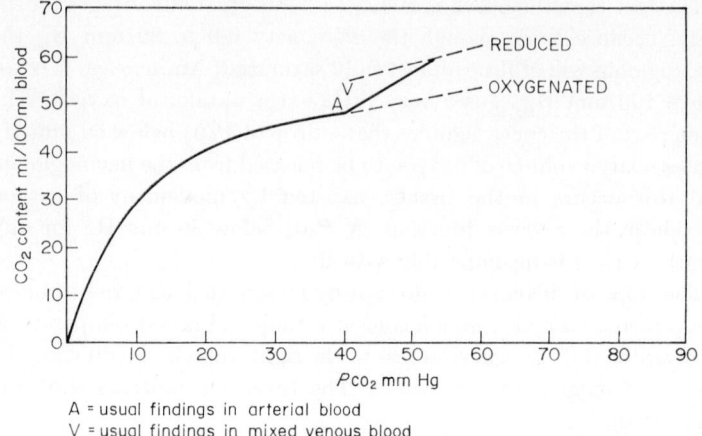

FIG. 6.2 CO_2 dissociation curve.

showing that larger volume changes occur for similar changes in tension than with oxygen. As most of the carbon dioxide in the blood is in the form of bicarbonate, any metabolic changes in the concentration of the latter alter the carbon dioxide dissociation curve. Metabolic acidosis lowers its position on the graph, and metabolic alkalosis raises it.

Body gas stores
Body stores of carbon dioxide are large, mainly as bicarbonate in tissue fluids, but the stores of oxygen are very small. If the volume of ventilation, or the composition of gases in the inspired air, alters, a new level of oxygen stores is reached in two minutes, whereas a new steady state for carbon dioxide is reached after fifteen to twenty minutes.

The ratio of $\dfrac{CO_2 \text{ produced}}{O_2 \text{ consumed}}$ is called the *respiratory quotient* (R.Q.). The normal value is 0·7 to 1·0 in fasting patients at rest.

SOME DIFFERENCES IN RESPIRATORY PHYSIOLOGY IN INFANTS

Infants cannot be regarded as small adults. They have a large surface area in relation to weight, and a high metabolic rate.

The airways have a greater relative diameter, and the anatomical

Respiratory Physiology

dead space is proportionally larger. The ribs are almost horizontal at rest, and inspiration cannot raise them much more. Therefore inspiration is mainly diaphragmatic, and anything which impedes diaphragmatic movement will cause respiratory distress.

These factors make respiration less efficient than in the adult, and an increase in alveolar ventilation is achieved by an increase in rate, which is expensive in terms of work, and needs a high oxygen intake.

Some comparative figures are shown in Table 6.2.

THE EFFECTS OF ADMINISTRATION OF HIGH OXYGEN CONCENTRATIONS

Oxygen should be administered to patients in concentrations just sufficient to cause maximal arterial saturation. Greater concentrations are unnecessary and may indeed be harmful.

In a patient with chronic hypoxia, whose respiratory centre does not respond to carbon dioxide, and who relies on the chemoreceptor reflex to maintain respiration, giving a high concentration of inspired oxygen may cause respiratory arrest. More commonly, it causes respiratory depression and a rising P_aCO_2.

If a healthy person breathes 100 per cent oxygen for 24 hours, substernal distress is experienced, and vital capacity is decreased. In animals, high inspired oxygen concentrations lead to death from pulmonary congestion and oedema. This does not occur with 50–60 per cent oxygen.

Pulmonary atelectasis may occur if the alveoli contain gas rich in oxygen, perhaps due to the greater solubility of this gas than nitrogen.

In premature babies, inhalation of high oxygen concentrations leads to retrolental fibroplasia, which may cause permanent blindness. Forty per cent oxygen is thought to be safe.

Anoxia

This term refers to a lack of oxygen in the whole or part of the body. Hypoxia is probably a better term, because a state completely without oxygen is incompatible with life. Hypoxaemia is the term which refers to desaturation of the arterial blood.

In acute hypoxia there is a cardiac and general body depression, leading after a time to cerebral and renal damage and death. There is a tendency for a metabolic acidosis to develop due to anaerobic

Table 6.2 (Adapted from Mushin). Variation of physiological data with age.

age	wt (Kg)	Ht (cm)	Total ventilation ml/min	rate/min	TV ml	Compliance ml/cm H_2O	resistance cm $H_2O/(L/sec)$
neonate	3	49	640	40	16	5	31
1 year	9	71	1500	30	50	10	30
8 years	25	125	4000	20	200	25	6
adult	66	171	8000	16	500	50	2

cellular metabolism. If the onset is more gradual, and hypoxia is chronic, compensatory changes occur, and a greater degree of hypoxaemia can be tolerated. These changes consist of polycythaemia, hyperventilation, tachycardia, and an increase in the density of the systematic capillary bed. All these factors increase the amount of oxygen available to the tissues. Finger clubbing often develops in such patients.

The degree of disability depends on the acuteness of onset, and also on the cause—for instance, a patient with congenital cyanotic heart disease may live reasonably comfortably with an oxygen saturation below 80 per cent whereas a patient with pulmonary emphysema may be acutely distressed with a saturation of 90 per cent. Part of the distress is due to mechanical difficulties of breathing.

Cyanosis may occur. This term refers only to a blue colour of the skin and mucous membranes, and has several causes. It may be due to hypoxia, either central, in which case there is associated hypoxaemia, or peripheral, due to stasis in the tissues, which may or may not be associated with arterial desaturation. On the other hand cyanosis may be due to the presence of abnormal pigments in the blood—sulphaemoglobin or methaemoglobin. A pink patient need not be well oxygenated, as is seen in carbon monoxide poisoning.

Cyanosis is noticeable when there is more than 5gm/100 ml of reduced haemoglobin in the arterial blood. It follows that if the patient's haemoglobin concentration is low enough, he cannot be cyanosed. In polycythaemia, cyanosis occurs readily. The presence of cyanosis is an unreliable sign of hypoxia, for the above reasons, and also because observers vary in their ability to detect the colour changes. The quality of the light may also be misleading.

The Causes of Hypoxia
1. anoxic—due to impaired oxygenation of the arterial blood.
    (i) reduced oxygen concentration in the inspired air
    (ii) inadequate alveolar ventilation
    (iii) impaired distribution or diffusion in the lungs
    (iv) venous to arterial shunts (in heart or lungs)
2. anaemic—due to the absence of sufficient functioning haemoglobin to maintain tissue oxygenation.
    Available O_2 = cardiac output × Hb conc^n. × per cent of saturation × 1·34.

3. stagnant—due to poor blood flow through the tissues.
4. histotoxic—due to poisoning of cellular enzymes.

The second, third and fourth of these are not necessarily associated with hypoxaemia, and can usually be recognised. If hypoxaemia is present, then the four varieties of anoxic anoxia must be differentiated. Reduced inspired oxygen concentration should be easily recognised. If diffusion is impaired, arterial saturation is usually normal at rest, but desaturation occurs on exercise.

If arterial desaturation is present at rest, the patient should be given 30 per cent oxygen to breathe. In the presence of a true venous to arterial shunt the blood will remain desaturated, but the saturation will rise almost to normal in patients with impaired alveolar ventilation, or with distribution problems. If there is maldistribution of inspired gas, the associated hyperventilation gives a lowered P_aCO_2 whereas alveolar hypoventilation, or respiratory failure, is associated with hypercarbia.

These tests, i.e. the response to exercise, the administration of 30 per cent oxygen, and the measurement of P_aCO_2, are easy to do, and form a basis for differential diagnosis. Many more sophisticated tests are available, and readers are referred to books on respiratory physiology.

The clinical signs of carbon dioxide retention are rather vague, and include tachycardia, raised blood pressure, sweating, warm extremities, confusion, restlessness and muscle twitching, leading eventually to coma. If respiratory failure is suspected, P_aCO_2 should be measured, and this may be used as a guide to the effectiveness of treatment. Various ventilation volumes may be measured, but children are not co-operative, and in any case it is hard to be accurate with small volumes. If the respiratory failure cannot be rapidly relieved by drugs, oxygen, and physiotherapy, then artificial ventilation should be instituted until the patient is again capable of maintaining his own ventilation adequately.

FURTHER READING

COMROE, J. H. et al. *The Lung*, 2nd Ed. 1962. Year Book Medical Publishers Inc.

CAMPBELL, E. J. M. et al. *Clinical Physiology*, 2nd Ed. 1963. Blackwell.

MUSHIN, W. W. Problems of Automatic Ventilation in Infants and Children 1962. *British Journal of Anaesthesia*, vol. **34**, 514.

CHAPTER

7

Cardiovascular Physiology

The heart may be regarded as a pump whose purpose is to supply the tissues with sufficient oxygenated blood so that the metabolic requirements of the cells are met under all circumstances. In fact, there are two pumps working in parallel, and the systems to be considered are the high resistance high pressure systemic circulation, and the low resistance low pressure pulmonary circulation.

THE HEART AS A PUMP

As with any other pump, the output is given by multiplying the volume ejected per stroke by the number of ejections per minute.

Cardiac output is thus the product of the *stroke volume* (which is the difference between the end diastolic volume and the end systolic volume q.v.) and the *heart rate*. The ventricles must pump blood from a low pressure venous system into a high pressure arterial system. However, the mode of action of the two ventricles differs in that the left ventricle has to propel blood into the high resistance systemic circuit, while the right ventricle ejects into the low resistance pulmonary vasculature; this difference in function is reflected in the anatomical arrangement of the muscle fibres of the two ventricles, the right being arranged to produce a volume pump, while the left is a pressure pump. The atria, being required to perform only little work, mainly existing as systemic and pulmonary venous reservoirs, have correspondingly thin muscular walls.

Actual ejection from the ventricles is preceded by the *isovolumetric contraction phase*, in which the ventricular volume does not change, but the heart becomes more spherical. During this time the atrioventricular valves close, and with further contraction of the ventricular muscle the pressure in the ventricles rises until the aortic and pulmonary valves open, when the rapid phase of systolic ejection takes place, in the early stage of which the ventricular pressure exceeds very slightly the pressure in the aorta or pulmonary artery. Rapid ejection is accompanied by distension of the aorta, and the output of blood into the aorta at first exceeds run-off into the distal vessels. As run-off and output equalise, the pressure in the aorta flattens off, and then reduced ejection from the ventricle begins, during which run-off from the aorta exceeds output from the ventricle and the pressure in the ventricle and aorta begins to fall. When the ventricles begin to relax, the aortic and pulmonary valves close due to the fall of ventricular pressure, and diastole begins with opening of the atrioventricular valves and ventricular filling.

Owing to the different mechanical structure of the two ventricles, and their different modes of action, left ventricular systole is completed fractionally sooner than right, and the closure of the aortic and pulmonary valves is asynchronous, accounting for the normal splitting of the pulmonary second sound on auscultation.

The volume of blood in the ventricle at the beginning of systole is termed the *end diastolic volume*, while that remaining when the valves close at the end of systole is called the *end systolic volume*.

Since cardiac output depends on stroke volume and heart rate, it can be varied by changes in either or both. If the stroke volume remains constant an increase in heart rate causes a directly proportional increase in cardiac output. This only applies at moderate increases of heart rate; at a rate of more than 150–160 beats per minute the filling time of the ventricles is so limited that the end diastolic volume, and therefore the stroke volume, is reduced. This limitation of cardiac output can occur at only slightly increased heart rates if sympathetic nerve action on the heart is interfered with by disease or drugs. Sympathetic nerve stimulation of the heart causes increased rate and myocardial contraction, with a decreased end systolic volume and therefore increased stroke volume, so that cardiac output rises.

Heart rate is influenced by a variety of factors, for example metabolic rate, exertion, emotional disturbance, hypovolaemia, age

Cardiovascular Physiology

etc. The metabolic rate itself will depend on such conditions as body temperature, the presence of infection, stress and endocrine disturbances. However, it is important to appreciate that changes in heart rate occur throughout early life and average values are given in Table 7.1. It is emphasized that these refer to resting conditions in normal subjects.

Table 7.1 Variation of heart rate with age.

Age	Heart rate
0–24 hours	125
1 day–1 week	140
1 week–3 months	160
3 months–1 year	150
1–3 years	130
3–8 years	100
8–12 years	90
12–16 years	80

The end diastolic volume is affected by the filling time (dependent on heart rate), the effective filling pressure and the distensibility of the ventricles. The filling pressure is the difference in pressure between the inside and the outside of the ventricles, and is thus dependent on the venous return and the negative intra-thoracic pressure. An increase of central venous pressure (q.v.) or an increase of negative intra-thoracic pressure (see Chapter 6) will produce an increased pressure gradient and so facilitate ventricular filling. At rapid heart rates, when filling time is reduced, atrial contraction becomes important in ventricular filling, although at normal rates it plays a minor role; thus atrial fibrillation does not cause a significant lowering of resting cardiac output but does interfere with the attainment of an effective output with exercise, so that exertion becomes limited.

The factors modifying ventricular distensibility in the normal heart are not well understood, but there is some evidence to suggest that catecholamines not only improve myocardial contraction but also the compliance of the ventricles.

The end systolic volume, the blood remaining in the ventricle after closure of the aortic or pulmonary valve, is dependent on the resistance against which the ventricle is pumping, and the force which the myocardium is exerting. If myocardial contractility is increased, either the end systolic volume will be decreased (so increasing stroke volume and cardiac output), or the vascular resistance will be increased so that the same volume of blood is ejected. In either case more work must be done by the heart.

Cardiac work is capable of measurement, being the product of the volume of fluid ejected and the pressure head. The left ventricular work is thus given by multiplying mean arterial pressure (q.v.) and cardiac output. The right and left ventricles pump equal volumes of blood, but the mean pulmonary artery pressure is only about one seventh of mean aortic pressure so that right ventricular work is only one seventh that of the left.

Cardiac work is dependent on aerobic metabolism of the myocardial muscle; increased work demands increased oxygen, and this is provided by increased coronary blood flow. The myocardium accounts for about 4 per cent of the cardiac output at rest, and coronary flow is directly related to oxygen consumption by the heart. Hypoxia can increase the coronary flow about five times, lowering of the myocardial Po_2 causing coronary arteriolar dilatation. The source of energy for cardiac contraction, as with skeletal muscle, is glucose, but the heart muscle can also use lactic acid released by anaerobic metabolism in the skeletal muscles and indeed, the utilization of lactic acid may exceed that of glucose. However, if the heart is hypoxic it will *produce* lactic acid as a metabolite.

Myocardial contractility depends on normal acid/base relationships and a normal electrolyte environment. Acidosis (whether metabolic or respiratory) causes a decrease of cardiac output and at a critical low pH cardiac arrest occurs, the heart stopping in a dilated state. A disturbed balance between potassium, sodium and calcium (see Chapter 4) can lead to serious interference with normal cardiac action.

Systemic Blood Pressure

The ejection of blood from the left ventricle into the systemic arterial system results in a pressure peak known as *systolic pressure*. Run-off of blood into the vascular bed causes a decline of pressure, and the lowest point reached during ventricular diastole is the *diastolic pressure*. The difference is the *pulse pressure*, and the average pressure attained in the system during the cardiac cycle is the *mean pressure*.

Cardiovascular Physiology

The mean pressure is *not* the arithmetic mean of systolic and diastolic pressure, but is obtained by dividing the area under a pressure curve by the width of the largest part of the curve (see Fig. 7.1). An approximate estimate of mean pressure can be obtained by adding together the diastolic pressure and one third of the pulse pressure. Mean pressure is important and has been called the functional pressure since it represents the *perfusion pressure*. Little change in mean pressure occurs in the larger arteries, but it falls moderately

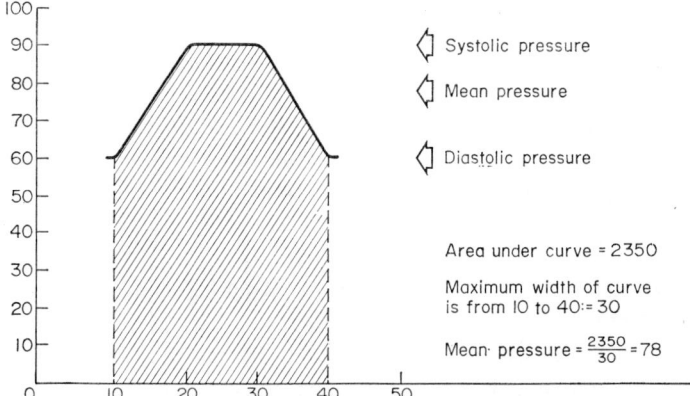

Fig. 7.1 Measurement of mean arterial pressures.

steeply as blood enters the small arteries while the gradient declines very steeply in the arterioles.

It is well known that hypertension occurs in most elderly persons, the characteristic feature being an increase of diastolic pressure due to loss of elasticity of the vessel walls. The 'normal' value of systolic/diastolic pressure of 120/70 mm Hg is not found in the early years of life, however, and average values for various age groups are given in Table 7.2.

The flow (Q) of fluid through a system of tubes obeys the pressure–resistance relationship shown in the equation:

$$Q = \frac{R}{P}$$

In other words the mean blood pressure in the arteries depends on the flow and the resistance in the system, or;

$$P = Q \times R$$

Table 7.2 Variation of systemic arterial pressure with age.

Age	S/D mm Hg
Newborn	80/45
1 year	95/65
2–8 years	100/65
9–10 years	105/65
11 years	110/70
12 years	115/70
13–14 years	120/70

The arterial system is one of increasing resistance from the large arteries to the periphery, because of the decreasing calibre of the vessels, and it is also capable of *change* in resistance because of the muscular nature of certain of the vessels and also due to sphincter mechanisms operating in the vascular tree.

In the present context flow depends on cardiac output, so we can re-write the equation:

Mean arterial pressure $\propto$ Cardiac output $\times$ Peripheral vascular resistance.

Thus increase in cardiac output (due to increased heart rate and/or stroke volume), without any change in vascular resistance, will cause an increase in mean pressure. Lowering of the cardiac output can be compensated for to some extent by increased vascular resistance (c.f. shock).

Changes in heart rate, peripheral vascular resistance and stroke volume, which would all affect mean pressure, must also modify systolic, diastolic and pulse pressure. The diastolic pressure is really a measurement of vascular resistance. An increase of vascular resistance causes difficulty of run-off of blood into the periphery, with retention of blood in the central vessels, so that both systolic and diastolic pressures rise, the increase of diastolic being relatively greater, with a reduction of pulse pressure. A decrease of resistance facilitates run-off with reduction of systolic and diastolic pressures, the diastolic lowering being relatively greater so that pulse pressure is increased.

An increase of heart rate occurring as in exercise would allow less time for run-off of blood into the periphery so that the diastolic pressure would rise and the pulse pressure decrease, but in fact a

Cardiovascular Physiology

compensatory vasodilatation occurs with a lowering of vascular resistance. In slowing of the heart, as in heart block, the diastolic pressure falls markedly due to increased run-off, and the pulse pressure widens.

If an increased stroke volume is ejected into the arterial system, the elastic vessels are stretched and the systolic pressure rises more than the diastolic so that the pulse pressure increases. A decreased stroke volume causes a lowering of systolic pressure, more marked than with the diastolic so that the pulse pressure falls.

The pressure in the small veins may be regarded as the amount of arterial pressure which is left after the passage of blood through the small arteries, arterioles and capillaries, this being about 20 cm of water (15 mm Hg). When the body is horizontal this venous pressure is quite adequate to return the blood to the heart, but in the upright position hydrostatic effects cause an increase of both mean arterial and venous pressure in the lower limbs and abdomen. The developing of excessively high venous pressures with pooling of blood and loss of fluid from the capillaries into the tissue spaces is prevented in the normal individual by arterial and venous vasomotor reflexes, the influence of respiration and the massaging effect of skeletal muscles. Loss of vasomotor tone has obvious consequences. Measurement of the peripheral venous pressure has little clinical importance, but the *central venous pressure*, that is, the pressure in the superior or inferior vena cava, gives useful information in patient management, because it reflects changes in blood volume and/or cardiac efficiency. Thus a high central venous pressure would indicate such states as low cardiac output and poor cardiac action, overloading of the circulation with blood or fluid, or cardiac tamponade.

The central venous pressure should be recorded from a fixed reference point, usually taken as the midpoint of the right atrium. The measurement of the pressure in the great veins in the thorax is complicated by the fact that the pressure is affected by the changes occurring in intrathoracic pressure during the respiratory cycle. Let us assume that the incoming venous pressure is 5 mm Hg, and that during quiet respiration the intrathoracic pressure during inspiration is -10 mm Hg, and in expiration it is -5 mm Hg. During inspiration the effective venous pressure is from 5 to -10, i.e., 15 mm Hg, while in expiration it is from 5 to -5, i.e. 10 mm Hg. Thus inspiration increases venous filling of the right atrium, and the effect is more marked with exercise when the inspiratory negative pressure is increased. On the other hand, artificial ventilation of the lungs by a positive pressure machine reverses the respiratory assistance to venous return as described in Chapter 9.

Pulmonary Blood Pressure

As already indicated, right ventricular work is only about one seventh that of the left, this being due to the fact that the pulmonary vascular resistance is considerably less than the systemic. As in the systemic circulation, conducting pulmonary arteries with a predominance of elastic tissue within their walls gradually merge into muscular arteries. In the systemic circulation the transition occurs in large arteries such as the common iliac, which conveys blood from a conducting vessel, the abdominal aorta, into a muscular artery, the femoral. The transition in the pulmonary circulation occurs in vessels of much smaller diameter, and although the muscular pulmonary arteries are similar to muscular systemic arteries in the presence of smooth muscle in the media, the wall is considerably thinner than in a systemic artery of comparable size so that the bore is correspondingly greater. In the adult the mean pulmonary artery pressure is about 15 mm Hg. The pressure in the pulmonary artery varies with respiration, being higher in expiration than inspiration. The variation is of the order of 3–6 mm Hg and corresponds to the pressure change in the pleural space to which reference has already been made.

Just as systemic venous pressure can be regarded as that amount of arterial blood pressure which is left after the blood has passed through the arterioles and capillaries, so pulmonary venous pressure represents the amount of pulmonary artery pressure left after perfusion of the lungs. However, the pulmonary venous pressure is more dependent on left heart action and is therefore more directly a function of left atrial pressure. The mean left atrial pressure is always slightly higher than the right. The pressure in the left atrium has important implications in the evaluation of pathological states in the heart and lungs; thus it enables a distinction to be made between the pulmonary hypertension due to obstruction of the mitral valve, and that due to intracardiac shunts.

In a normal person at rest only a fraction of the pulmonary capillaries is perfused at any given time. Moreover, blood flow in the

Cardiovascular Physiology

lungs tends to follow a gravitational path so that most of the blood is distributed to the dependent parts of the lungs (air flow is similarly distributed).

The whole of the cardiac output must pass through the lungs as these are situated between the right and left sides of the heart. Pulmonary artery pressure remains fairly constant over a wide range of pulmonary blood flows. The volume of blood in the lungs and left atrium is between 10 per cent and 20 per cent of the total blood volume. The relationship between pulmonary blood flow and mean pulmonary artery pressure is curvilinear, but the early part of the curve is almost linear with a very gradual ascent, so that considerable increases in cardiac output are accompanied by very small increases in mean pulmonary artery pressure, as shown in Fig. 7.2. In

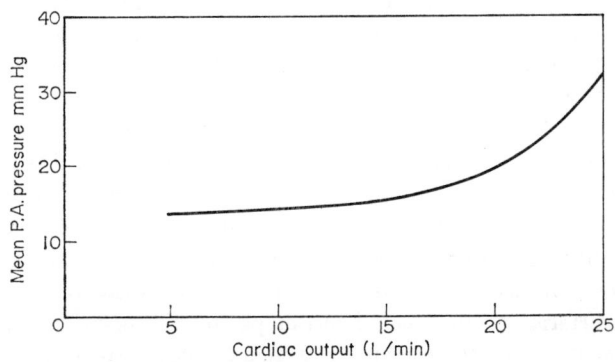

FIG. 7.2 Relationship between pulmonary artery pressure and blood flow.

congenital heart disease, however, increases in pulmonary blood flow due to shunts may be accompanied by considerable increases in pressure (q.v. Chapter 14).

In the normal subject as cardiac output increases as a result of exercise, pulmonary vascular resistance falls owing to passive distension of the pulmonary vessels, and an increase in the number of capillaries perfused by blood occurs, so that all areas of the lungs are being utilised and blood distribution within the lungs is no longer preferentially influenced by gravity.

In haemodynamic evaluation of a patient the pulmonary wedge pressure is frequently measured, by impacting a cardiac catheter into one of the smaller pulmonary arteriolar branches well out in the lung. This gives an *estimate* of the pulmonary venous or left atrial pressure and is of use in calculating the resistance to flow imposed by the pulmonary circulation, according to the equation:

$$\text{Pulmonary vascular resistance in dynes sec cm}^{-5} = \frac{(\text{Mean P.A. Pressure} - \text{Mean Wedge Pressure}) \text{ mm Hg} \times 80}{\text{Pulmonary blood flow (L/min)}}$$

The normal resistance is about 100 dynes sec cm^{-5} and in certain pathological conditions it may be twenty times as great as this.

The Circulation in the Newborn

In the foetus the two ventricles work together as systemic pumps, driving blood from the great veins mainly into the aorta. The placenta and foetal tissues are all supplied with arterial blood providing a parallel network of vessels between the arteries and the veins. The right and left sides of the heart are linked via the foramen ovale and the ductus arteriosus. The inferior vena caval blood stream (carrying with it the oxygenated blood from the umbilical vein) splits into two streams in the right atrium, the major portion passing via the foramen ovale, while the remainder joins with the superior vena cava and coronary sinus blood to enter the right ventricle. The left atrial blood enters the left ventricle to be pumped into the aorta. The right ventricular blood is also pumped into the aorta via the ductus arteriosus, only a small portion passing through the lungs, this being achieved by the presence of a high resistance to flow. The high resistance in the lungs is partly due to their collapsed state in utero, and partly to the fact that the foetal pulmonary arteries resemble their systemic counterpart, the muscular pulmonary arteries being thickwalled and of small bore.

It is of interest to compare the relative blood flows through various parts of the foetal circulation. About 55 per cent of the combined output of both ventricles passes through the placenta, which is a low resistance circuit in parallel with the foetal tissues. Only 12 per cent of the output passes through the lungs owing to the high resistance. The foramen ovale carries 46 per cent and the ductus arteriosus 30 per cent of the flow.

It is also instructive to examine the oxygen saturations in the foetus. That in the umbilical vein is about 80 per cent, but admixture with venous blood from the portal vein, lower half of the body and

Cardiovascular Physiology

lungs reduces this to 65 per cent by the time the blood has reached the left ventricle, ascending aorta and aortic arch. Further mixture of desaturated blood reaching the aorta from the right ventricle via the ductus arteriosus reduces the oxygen saturation in the descending aorta to 58 per cent. The tissues of the foetus are thus all supplied with blood at approximately the same Po_2, which is only about one third of that of an adult, a situation which has been described as the 'Mount Everest in utero', and accounts for the higher than normal haemoglobin found in the newborn.

After birth, with the establishment of respiration, the pulmonary vascular resistance falls due to the inflation of the lungs and presumably the straightening out of the compressed alveolar capillaries, but the resistance is still higher than in the older infant due to the presence of the thick-walled muscular arteries. The fall of resistance is sufficient to produce a significant reduction of pulmonary artery pressure which is now below systemic. The establishment of increased pulmonary blood flow results in the left atrial pressure slightly exceeding that in the right, so that the foramen ovale closes, at first functionally and later anatomically. The ductus arteriosus remains open for several days after birth and the flow is now intermittently from aorta to pulmonary artery.

During the first months of life the thick walled muscular pulmonary arteries gradually become thinner walled, with a further decrease in resistance to flow, the process being termed *involution*. The change from the high resistance pulmonary circulation to low resistance is accompanied by a correspondingly lessened amount of work performed by the right ventricle, so that the wall of the ventricle becomes thinner and its compliance increases.

The above features of the foetal circulation have implications in the management of congenital heart disease, which will be considered in Chapter 14.

The changes occurring in the circulation of the child are shown in Table 7.3.

The Control of the Circulation

The regular rhythmical beat of the heart is an inherent property of cardiac muscle, and the rate is normally set by the sino-atrial node pacemaker, conduction of impulses generated by the node taking place through the wall of the right atrium to the atrio-ventricular node and thence to the atrio-ventricular bundle of His, with its right and left branches. The atrio-ventricular node consists of an upper atrio-nodal region, a nodal area, and a nodal-His area. Under certain circumstances clinical 'nodal' rhythms are seen probably arising from cells between the nodal-His area and the bundle itself.

Table 7.3 Pressure changes in the circulation with age.

Pressures mm Hg	Newborn	Infants & Children
Right atrium	Mean 0–3	1–5
Right ventricle	35–65/1–5	15–30/2–5
Pulmonary artery	35–65/20–40	15–30/5–10
	mean 25–40	mean 10–20
Pulmonary wedge	—	mean 5–12
Left atrium	mean 1–4	mean 5–10
Left ventricle	80/3–5	80–130/5–10

The cardiac output depends on heart rate, filling pressure, distensibility and contractility. The heart rate is modified mainly by the action of the vagus and sympathetic nerves on the pacemaker, and to a minor degree by catecholamine release from the adrenal medulla, and such modification depends on sensory information being received by the cardiovascular centres in the brain. The medulla contains nerve cells responsible for vaso-constriction, cardio-stimulation and cardio-inhibition. The hypothalamus is concerned in the distribution of blood for the control of body temperature, so that a drop of body temperature causes a decrease in heart rate, while an increase of temperature causes a tachycardia. Hypothalamic lesions may prevent the body adjusting to environmental conditions, because sweating and cutaneous vasodilation or vasoconstriction no longer occur in response to the appropriate stimuli.

Pressure and Stretch Receptors

Systemic arterial pressure is monitored mainly by pressoreceptors situated in the carotid sinus, common carotid arteries and arch of the aorta. Other receptors are situated along the thoracic and mesenteric arteries. The pressoreceptors are continuously discharging impulses to the cardiovascular centres in the brain, but the rate of discharge responds to increase of pressure, so that a burst of dis-

Cardiovascular Physiology

discharges occurs with each pressure pulse. A continuously high arterial pressure results in greatly increased afferent impulses with stimulation of the cardio-inhibitor centre and vagal slowing of the heart, a decrease in cardiac contractility, and peripheral vasodilatation. Pulse pressure is important in determining the rate of firing of the pressoreceptors. Thus a reduction of pulse pressure, with no change in mean arterial pressure, decreases the stimulation of the cardio-inhibitor centre and therefore promotes increased heart rate, increased cardiac contraction and peripheral vasoconstriction. It is of course well known that digital pressure over the carotid arteries can result in profound hypotension.

Stretching of the right atrium and great veins causes afferent impulses to stimulate the cardio-stimulator centre resulting in increased heart rate (Bainbridge reflex). Similar receptors in the left atrium respond to stretching by causing an increased urine flow and therefore a reduction of blood volume, but the exact mechanism is unknown.

There are pressoreceptors in the pulmonary arteries responding in the same way as the systemic ones but to a much less extent, which is reasonable in view of the small pressure changes normally occurring in the pulmonary circulation.

Chemoreceptors

These sensors are situated in the carotid and aortic bodies near the carotid sinus and in the aortic arch. The nerve endings are sensitive to a decrease in Po_2, an increase of Pco_2 and a decrease of pH. Stimulation of the chemoreceptors does not affect the heart rate, but chiefly affects pulmonary ventilation causing an increase in rate and depth. There is an indirect effect on systemic blood pressure which rises due to peripheral vasoconstriction.

Neural and Hormonal Control of the Cardiovascular System

The vagus nerve releases acetyl choline and stimulation of the vagus results in bradycardia. The sympathetic (cardio-accelerator) nerves to the heart release nor-adrenaline resulting in tachycardia and increased myocardial contractility.

The actions of adrenaline and nor-adrenaline on the heart and blood vessels are important in that although both are sympathomimetic agents there are differences in their actions. It is postulated that the heart and smooth muscle contain alpha- and beta-adrenergic receptors. Alpha-receptor stimulation results in increased permeability of the cell membrane to sodium ions, and the resulting depolarization causes contraction of smooth muscle (in the case of blood vessels, therefore, vasoconstriction). This is the so-called direct action of adrenaline. Beta-adrenergic receptor stimulation increases cell metabolism, speeds the sodium pump and so increases polarization, so that smooth muscle relaxes (e.g. small intestine, or peripheral vasodilatation)—the so called metabolic effect of adrenaline.

Whereas the sympathetic nerves release nor-adrenaline (apart from some which release acetyl choline), the adrenal medulla liberates adrenaline with some nor-adrenaline. Nor-adrenaline, adrenaline and iso prenaline as a class are called catecholamines. The *net* action of a particular agent on a particular tissue or organ depends on whether stimulation of alpha-adrenergic or beta-adrenergic receptors dominates. Moreover, the cutaneous blood vessels, those in the skeletal muscles, and the coronary arteries may respond in different ways. In so far as the heart is concerned one must distinguish between the *chronotropic* effect (rate) and the *inotropic* effect (contractility) both of which depend on beta-receptor stimulation.

Alpha-receptors can be blocked by drugs such as phentolamine and phenoxybenamine while beta-receptors are blocked by propranalol.

Adrenaline acts on the heart by stimulating the beta-receptors so that heart rate and contractility are increased. The vascular effects are usually cutaneous vasoconstriction, with dilatation of the arterioles in skeletal muscle. In large doses the alpha-receptor effects dominate so that a pressor response to adrenaline occurs; however, when small doses of adrenaline are administered peripheral vasodilatation can occur due to beta-receptor stimulation, so much so that hypotension results despite the inotropic and chronotropic effects leading to increased cardiac output.

The cardiovascular effects of nor-adrenaline are the result of stimulation of alpha- and beta-receptors in the heart and the resistance blood vessels, with a marked predominance of the alpha-action. Force of cardiac contraction is increased, and alpha-receptor effects on resistance vessels cause profound vasoconstriction, which can only be abolished by large doses of alpha-blocking agents. A reflex bradycardia is found unless the vagus is blocked with atropine.

Both adrenaline and nor-adrenaline cause renal artery constriction with impairment of renal blood flow; this is an important consideration in post-operative care.

Isoprenaline is mainly a beta-adrenergic stimulator. It therefore produces increased myocardial contraction, and increased heart rate so increasing cardiac output. It also produces peripheral vasodilatation.

The coronary blood vessels contain alpha-receptors mediating vasoconstriction and beta-receptors mediating vasodilatation. Beta-adrenergic blockade will allow catecholamines to produce vasoconstriction of the coronary arteries and this has important implications in the management of patients with heart disease and arrhythmias.

Blood Flow, Microcirculation and Organ Perfusion

The rate of flow of fluid through a tube depends on the driving pressure and the resistance to flow. If the pressure increases the flow increases, while if the resistance increases the flow decreases. This is expressed in the equation.

$$\text{Flow} = \frac{\text{Pressure gradient}}{\text{Resistance}}$$

In the case of a tissue vascular bed the pressure gradient is the arterial pressure minus the venous pressure, and the resistance is mainly determined by the calibre of the arterioles, this being dependent on the vasomotor tone.

The resistance to flow is not only determined by the vessel calibre, however, and in any event is not in direct relationship to the cross-section area. In the case of a simple fluid it is assumed that the fluid consists of layers which slide one upon the other; the layer adjacent to the vessel wall is barely moving, while, going towards the centre of the vessel, the velocity of flow increases rapidly at first and then more slowly to reach a maximum value at the centre. Such is called a Newtonian fluid, and obeys Poiseuille's equation, which states that the flow is directly proportional to the pressure gradient and the fourth power of the radius, and inversely proportional to the length of the vessel and the viscosity of the fluid. Owing to the fact that flow is a function of the fourth power of the radius a small increase in calibre of a vessel will allow a much greater increase in flow. Thus an increase in radius of an arteriole of about 20 per cent will increase flow by 100 per cent with the same pressure gradient.

For a Newtonian fluid flow is directly proportional to the pressure gradient, and the relationship will be linear as shown in A, Fig. 7.3.

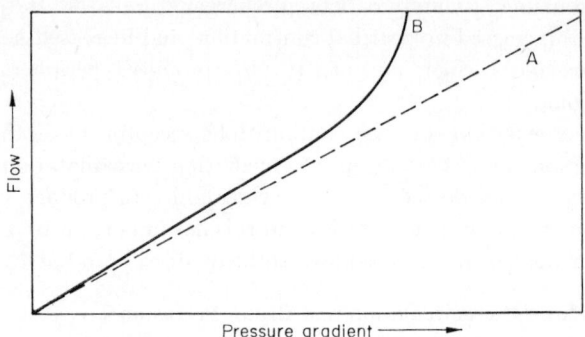

FIG. 7.3 Relation between pressure gradient and flow for a Newtonian fluid (A) and blood (B).

In the case of blood the relationship is curvilinear (B), and there are two main reasons for this. Firstly, blood is not a Newtonian fluid of constant viscosity, but consists of cells suspended in plasma, the cells tending to be aggregated towards the centre of the stream in small vessels. In large vessels the viscosity of blood is not dependent on the size of the tube, but as the calibre decreases and streaming of the cells takes place towards the centre of the vessels, the viscosity decreases, the peripheral layer of plasma acting as a lubricant. Secondly, the blood vessels are not rigid tubes; the vessel walls stretch during cardiac systole, and the distending force causing the vessels to expand must be balanced by a restraining force, due to the tension of the fibres in the vessel walls. Owing to this distension of the vessel walls during systole, a greater flow is possible than with tubes of fixed calibre.

The viscosity of blood depends on the number of cells suspended within it, being considerably increased in polycythaemia. It also depends on temperature, the viscosity increasing with decreased temperature. When blood flow is low, as in low cardiac output states, the red blood cells clump together to form rouleaux resulting in increased viscosity.

Cardiovascular Physiology

The blood vessels can be divided into *resistance vessels* and *capacitance vessels* with regard to function. Resistance to flow is of course shown by any vessel, but variation in resistance largely occurs in the arterioles. Capacitance vessels are those in which blood can collect (and sometimes pool) and these are mainly the veins.

The resistance to flow through the systemic vasculature is called the *total peripheral resistance* and can be calculated according to the equation:

$$\text{Total peripheral resistance dynes sec cm}^{-5} = \frac{(\text{Mean aortic pressure} - \text{mean central venous pressure}) \text{ mm Hg} \times 80}{\text{systemic blood flow (L/min)}}$$

The function of blood vessels is to transport blood to and from the tissues, in order to allow tissue respiration to take place, and to remove products of metabolism from the cells. The tissues, from the point of view of the circulation, are composed of large numbers of microcirculatory units. Each unit consists of arterioles, terminal arterioles, capillaries and venules, and the vessels are arranged both in series and in parallel. Within the unit blood flow can be regulated by pre-capillary sphincters situated at the junction of the terminal arterioles with the capillary network and post-capillary sphincters where the network joins the venules. Resistance to flow through the unit is set by the calibre of the arterioles and the tone of the pre-capillary sphincters.

Certain vessels within a microcirculatory unit can act as a bypass, allowing blood to flow from arteriole to venule without passing through the capillary network, and such a shunt vessel is utilized by shutting down the pre-capillary sphincters to other parts of the unit. Tissue exchange of ions, gases and metabolites occurs chiefly across the capillary walls and venules. Transcapillary exchange of fluid is dependent on the pressure gradient between the capillary and tissue spaces and the osmotic differences between the plasma and the interstitial fluid. In certain conditions increased capillary permeability leads to loss of fluid from the vascular compartment into the interstitial compartment, and consequent reduction of plasma volume.

The output of blood from the left ventricle is used to perfuse various tissues which are arranged in parallel, excluding the hepatic portal circulation. The *distribution* of blood to various organs and tissues is thus dependent on the relative vascular resistance in the various areas. That there is a preferential distribution of blood is obvious when considering the pathological state of shock, where the cutaneous network and the limbs are poorly perfused in order to achieve better perfusion of more vital areas. The factors affecting the distribution of blood to various organs are complex and beyond the scope of the present work.

CHAPTER

8

Patient Monitoring

The purpose of this chapter is to outline the principles and pitfalls of monitoring in a paediatric I.T.U. rather than to give a detailed description of the techniques of electromechanical instrumentation in infants and children. The purpose of monitoring is to increase patient safety while not impeding treatment or compromising sterility. A monitoring system is one used to warn of risk to the patient in the acute sense, or in the long term to warn of change in the patient whether progressive or retrogressive.

The system of monitoring may or may not involve instrumentation. To be of maximum value it should meet the following criteria:
1. It should be easy to apply
2. It should be safe to apply to the patient
3. It should be easy to operate
4. It should be safe to operate
5. It should be worthwhile
6. It should be able to produce a permanent record as needed
7. It should be virtually indestructible, for many instruments seem designed with ease of destruction in mind, while many operators take on the contest of destruction of the seemingly indestructible with the greatest dedication.

PURCHASE OF INSTRUMENTS

Finance is the all important consideration in instrumentation. The limitation set by lack of funds soon defeats the aspirations of the keenest clinician. Instrument systems are only as good as their components. The higher the quality of the components the greater is the price. Fortunately this rise of price is usually accompanied by increased accuracy of performance together with greater reliability. Higher price does not mean that if sufficient is paid then perfection is achieved. All electronic equipment is fallible, and much extra money will be expended if many 'fail safe' mechanisms are incorporated. Equipment requires expert technical servicing on a regular basis, and to embark on a monitoring programme without such help is foolhardy and wasteful. Above all, it must be remembered that, as with all apparatus, it has a life expectancy after which, although it can be kept going, it is questionable whether in terms of its inefficiency it can be allowed to carry on in service.

Consideration of the precise needs of the monitoring programme must be made before purchase is contemplated. Advice should be sought from independent sources as to the applicability of the desired instruments to the requirements in mind, and reasonably long term trial of systems is desirable. Delay to allow trial and contemplation at the pre-purchase stage may well save much frustration later.

THE PAEDIATRIC I.T.U. AND MONITORING

The patients admitted to a paediatric I.T.U. will be those that are admitted to a children's hospital. This means that children from the first day of life to those in their fourteenth year will be met. Monitoring of the older child is not unlike that of the adult. We will thus be considering the problems in monitoring the younger age group in particular. Monitoring may be classed into two types:

(a) Continuous or semi-continuous monitoring
(b) Intermittent monitoring.

The nursing staff are well suited to carry out the first type of monitoring while the medical staff due to their many other commitments subscribe far better to the latter.

A plea has been made for centralised monitoring in the adult I.T.U., as it saves duplication of equipment, allows more frequent observation of individual patients, it reduces patient disturbance and frees staff for other duties. If centralised monitoring in a paediatric I.T.U. takes the nurse from the vicinity of the patient, it threatens disaster. The sick child needs to be monitored, but also requires someone constantly at the cot or incubator side to supervise. Changes in the clinical condition of a sick child can occur with alarming speed and are often unheralded, so that there is no time to see if it is the monitoring equipment or the patient that has had cessation of function. It is essential therefore that treatment can be effected by the nurse already standing at the bedside.

The stress of monitoring is thus laid on the nursing staff. Given encouragement, nurses quickly gain experience in the use of the apparatus and may eventually carry out the minor servicing procedures on these machines. There is no place for occasional use of machinery by either nursing or medical staff. Only by constant careful practice of any monitoring technique can consistency of meaningful results be obtained. Careful application and use will give good results, but this must be followed by circumspect interpretation.

The systems of monitoring to be employed will essentially be made up of four components, a detector, a transducer, an amplifier and a display system. The detector is necessary to collect the physiological signal. The transducer changes the form of energy in this signal to one which may be increased in power and eventually displayed. In electronic monitoring, the transducer converts the physiological signal into an electric current which is then amplified and eventually displayed on an oscilloscope screen. To this may be added a permanent recording system. This may be an ink record on paper, a tracing on heat-sensitive paper, or ultra-violet recording or the use of magnetic tape. A permanent record allows reference at a future time, and thus gives greater certainty about changes that have taken place than is possible using the transient display system.

Blood Pressure

Measurement of the blood pressure has considerable importance in patient monitoring, but interpretation of the results obtained must be tempered by consideration of the state of the vascular bed before assumptions are made in respect of cardiac function.

Indirect measurement

Estimation of the arterial pressure by use of a brachial occlusive cuff and radial artery palpation is well known. It is important for accuracy of measurement that the cuff be of the correct size; too narrow a cuff causes a high reading to be obtained and too wide a cuff causes a low reading. The cuff width should ideally be 20 per cent greater than the circumference of the extremity to which it is applied. It is thus important to have a variety of sizes of cuff for the patients in a paediatric I.T.U. A 2·5 cm wide cuff is suitable for the first year of life rising to a 9 cm cuff in the 4–8 year olds; a 6 cm cuff is available for those in between, while for larger patients an adult cuff suffices. Folding an adult cuff under no circumstances will provide accurate recordings. The rate of cuff deflation is important if an accurate measurement is to be made and should not exceed 5 mm/sec.

Application of a stethoscope over the artery distal to the occlusive cuff during deflation allows a series of sounds to be heard. The onset of the sounds marks the systolic point, whereas the commencement of muffling or abrupt fading marks the diastolic pressure. Auscultatory determination of the diastolic pressure is liable to considerable inaccuracy; in infants both the systolic and the diastolic points may be difficult to ascertain and this is particularly true in neonates and patients with low blood pressures. Palpation determination of systolic pressure in infants offers similar difficulties; when the blood pressure is low and accurate determination is most required it is then most difficult to measure.

Double cuff techniques using an oscillotonometer, although achieving success and popularity in adults, do not seem to be useful in small children in spite of special small cuffs.

The 'flush technique', involving emptying the limb of blood and applying the occlusive cuff at a pressure above the expected systolic, and then watching for the appearance of a flush during deflation, works well in the healthy child but in the hypotensive critically ill patient gives unreliable results.

Electrical methods of detection of the reappearance of the pulse wave distal to the occlusive cuff seem to be poorer in small children than adults and poorest when the blood pressure is low.

Direct measurement
In the face of so many difficulties using indirect measurement, direct measurement, when accurate knowledge of blood pressure is required, is the only answer.

Arterial cannulae are best introduced by percutaneous puncture even in small children. In the larger child the radial artery is satisfactory while in the very small child femoral puncture is attended with few sequelae provided a small cannula is used. Small bore disposable cannulae seem satisfactory for the technique, and the introduction is often facilitated by passing a nylon guide proximally up the vessel after the metal stillette has been removed. Provided that care is taken to maintain cannula patency, blood pressure may be recorded for several days.

Detection, transduction, amplification and display of the wave form cause no great difficulty. The connecting tube from the cannula to the detector-transducer is of importance, because too wide a tube and inertia of the fluid mass produce difficulties, too narrow a tube causes a difficulty with friction, while too long a connecting tube leads to exaggeration of the problems. The response of the system is dependent not only on the transducer but upon careful attention to the fluid coupling and the absence of air bubbles from it. These problems become exaggerated in small children as the energy production in attaining any blood pressure is less, but the energy loss in the fluid coupling tends to be constant as it is not reduced in size for small patients.

The ideal system involves getting rid of the fluid coupling, that is, catheter-tip transduction. Here the transducer and the detector are both at the intravascular site at which the pressure is to be measured. This largely does away with the problem of arranging that the level of the membrane of the transducer is at the same level as the site at which it is desired to measure the pressure in the patient. Catheter transducers are available, but the perfect instrument giving good constant results with facilities for blood sampling even in small patients at the present time awaits manufacture.

Direct monitoring offers the only continuous method of display of blood pressure. It is more difficult than indirect monitoring and has a potential morbidity not present in the indirect method. It is the only realistic method available for monitoring blood pressure for procedures such as cardio-pulmonary bypass and the immediate after care of cardiac patients, and also for procedures involving large changes in blood volume or of blood pressure such as the removal of a phaeochromocytoma.

Central venous pressure
The veins may be regarded as the sump of the cardiovascular system.

The measurement of the pressure in the central veins reflects the effective fluid content of the sump. It cannot however be taken as an isolated measurement but must be considered in conjunction with the arterial pressure and general clinical state of the patient. The *trend* of venous pressure is of considerably greater importance than an isolated measurement.

Venous cannulae are inserted via suitable routes into either the superior or inferior vena cava. Cannulation of the inferior vena cava is said to have a higher incidence of thromboembolic sequelae than the superior route. Cannulation of peripheral veins *per se* is not satisfactory as pressure recordings within them do not accurately reflect central venous pressure. Introduction of a catheter into a peripheral vein may be effected by percutaneous puncture using an appliance such as 'Intracath',* but is better effected using the 'E.Z.'* type of catheter where the catheter itself is the largest component to be passed into the vessel; the catheter is then threaded to the great veins. Entry is best gained to the superior vena cava by use of the antecubital veins or brachial basilic vein; the catheter is gradually advanced and the correct position is shown by a good respiratory swing on either the saline manometer or the oscilloscope trace, and is confirmed by the easy introduction and withdrawal of fluid. Some idea of the length of catheter that has been introduced can be obtained by comparing the catheter length with the simulated route of introduction externally on the patient, thus avoiding accidental atrial or ventricular positioning. Entry from the brachial cephalic vein to the superior cava is far more difficult, the catheter often being held up at the point of passage from the superficial to the deep system. The external jugular route can also be used.

Unfortunately in small children large peripheral veins in the arms and neck are not often in evidence. Entry to the subclavian veins by supra- or infra-clavicular puncture has been used. Unfortunately both carry the risk of pneumothorax. Percutaneous catheterisation of the internal jugular vein lying beneath the sternomastoid muscle offers a simple safe route in small patients. This procedure may be carried out whether the vessel is palpable or not, and the technique lends itself to safe use in even the smallest child.

It is important that the measurements of pressure made are always

---

* Manufactured by Deseret Pharmaceutical Co., Sandy, Utah, U.S.A.

referred to the same level, that is, the mid right atrium. It is presumed that the catheter introduced gives a continuous column of fluid from the right atrium to the detector membrane of the transducer. To give a correct reading, therefore, the membrane level must be the same as the level at which the reading is presumed to be taken. If the detector membrane is above the desired reference point the effect is that of a column of liquid hanging on the membrane and a low reading results; if the membrane is below then a high reading results. A simple system of arranging the levels of the manometers is thus desirable.

If a rapid response in venous manometry is not necessary, the saline manometer gives a satisfactory measurement of central venous pressure. If rapid response is required (as in cardio-pulmonary bypass surgery) electronic manometry is preferable. Accurate blood replacement during major surgery in small children is probably better controlled using central venous pressure measurement in addition to arterial pressure recordings.

The Electrocardiogram

All muscle when actively contracting has associated electrical charges. The recording of these charges constitutes the object of electrocardiography. The currents produced by heart muscle activity are transmitted through the body tissues and fluid to the skin and can be detected by suitably placed electrodes. It must be stressed at all times that the E.C.G. gives no information in respect of the mechanical and hydraulic ability of the heart. The E.C.G. does not tell the observer if the patient is alive; only by observation of pulse and blood pressure and resultant perfusion in conjunction with the E.C.G. can one be sure of this. Not infrequently in small children one can see an E.C.G. rhythm changing to ventricular fibrillation and again reverting back to regular complexes in a child who is clinically dead, there being no cardiac output to support life.

Care must be taken in the attachment of electrodes to patients, as loose or dry plates lead to abnormal recordings. Particularly in small children self adhesive electrodes are simpler and satisfactory, and are preferred to the metal plate with a rubber band holding it on the limb. If sequential precordial electrodes are used in small children care must be taken to ensure that the conductive jelly from one recording site does not interfere with the next or the result will be that of a common electrode. No single lead will display all the information obtained by electrocardiography. The greatest nuisances of electrocardiography are artefacts. These must be distinguished from proper meaningful signals or misdiagnosis may occur. Drying of the electrode jelly allows the base line to wander slowly; 50 cycle interference causes a wide base line, the peaks of the QRS complex usually showing over the top. This can usually be minimised by adequate earthing. Use of electric blankets for heating the patient leaves him in a bath of 50 cycle activity and little can be done except to switch off the blanket in order to display the E.C.G. trace. Disconnection of a patient lead gives rise to a straight line which can be confused with asystole. Muscle tremor usually spreads and obscures the base line, but this spread is much coarser and more irregular than that caused by 50 cycle interference. Patient movement, active or passive, causes the trace to leap about in an irregular fashion so that the normal complexes are lost and ventricular fibrillation may be simulated.

Detailed consideration of the E.C.G. and its abnormalities can be found in any of the many reference texts on this subject. Only a superficial survey of the method of observation and of the abnormalities seen will be considered.

The first wave on a normal E.C.G. trace is the P wave; this is usually an upward deflection and represents depolarisation of the atria. The second wave, a combination of three, constitutes the QRS complex representing the depolarisation of the ventricles. The third wave—the T wave—represents repolarisation of the ventricles. Repolarisation of the atria is not observed as the wave form is buried in the QRS complex, this occurring during ventricular contraction. The P–R interval is measured from the beginning of the P wave to the beginning of the R wave. It represents the time for conduction of the impulse, which is to set off ventricular contraction, from its origin in the sinus node to its arrival at the ventricles. It should, in health, not exceed 0·2 sec, usually the interval is 0·16–0·18 sec, but in children it may be shorter, 0·12–0·14 sec. The main abnormality of the P–R interval is its prolongation in heart block. The Q wave is a downward deflection, often absent, the R being an upward deflection followed by the S wave which is downward. These three, the QRS complex, should be considered together; their duration should

Patient Monitoring

not exceed 0·12 sec. The T wave is normally upward except occasionally in lead III. The S–T segment should be on the isoelectric line.

Abnormalities of the E.C.G. trace may be found as deviations of rate, rhythm, 'complex', interval times and electrical distribution about the isoelectric line.

Both during and after intrathoracic operations children not infrequently show E.C.G. abnormalities. These changes may be induced by manual or mechanical manipulation of the heart or of the great vessels, hypoxia or hypercapnia, and disturbances of electrolytes. Intrapericardial drains during the postoperative period may also cause irregularities. Fortunately the majority of abnormalities observed are transient and thus of no clinical significance. The abnormalities only become of significance when they persist and interfere with cardiac output and tissue perfusion or act as a herald of more dangerous changes to follow.

Both increase and decrease of heart rate can cause a fall of cardiac output as described in Chapter 7. In sinus tachycardia, the heart rate is rapid; there is a normal but rapid E.C.G. trace. Paroxysmal atrial tachycardia produces a characteristic tracing and if unrelieved can result in heart failure. Atrial fibrillation and atrial flutter both lead to heart failure; the atrial rates are rapid and the ventricles cannot thus respond to all the stimuli offered. In fibrillation the ventricular rate though rapid, but much slower than that of the atria, is grossly irregular. The E.C.G. shows absence of any regular P waves in the standard leads. On the other hand in atrial flutter the ventricular rate is often regular but there is a response only to every second, third or fourth atrial beat. The E.C.G. shows the picture of rapid regular atrial activity but with abnormal P waves. In both atrial flutter and fibrillation the atrial contraction is not only rapid but is ineffective as far as the final filling of the ventricles is concerned. Arrhythmias are treated as described in Chapter 14. Typical traces are shown in Fig. 8.1.

Ventricular tachycardia may occur as a primary event; it rapidly leads to heart failure if untreated. Unifocal ventricular tachycardia is characterised by rapidly occurring QRS complexes of regular though abnormal shape at regular intervals. Multifocal ventricular tachycardia has rapidly occurring QRS complexes of varying size and shape. P waves are not in evidence in either rhythm. Both may be precursors of ventricular fibrillation.

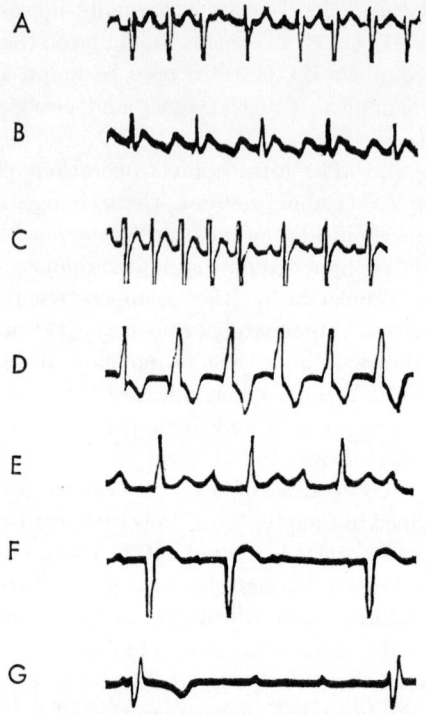

FIG. 8.1 Some abnormalities of the electrocardiogram.

A *Atrial fibrillation* Irregularly irregular, atrial rate 350–600/min, ventricular rate 120/min.
B *Atrial flutter* 2:1 block, atrial rate 200–400/min, ventricular rate 110/min.
C *Atrial tachycardia* Regular rapid ventricular rate, last 3 complexes show sinus rhythm.
D *Ventricular tachycardia* Bizarre large ventricular complexes.
E *1st degree heart block* P–R interval more than 0·2 sec.
F *2nd degree heart block* Increased P–R interval until a beat is dropped.
G *3rd degree heart block* Complete A–V dissociation, atrial rate 70–80/min, ventricular rate 20–40/min.

Ventricular fibrillation is associated with absence of cardiac output. The E.C.G. is characterised by bizarre irregular complexes. Rapid restoration of the circulation is necessary or the condition becomes irreversible.

Deviation of the S–T segment from the isoelectric line will be seen if hypoxia is present, and the deviation will return to normal when this state has been corrected unless the hypoxia has been severe and prolonged. In hyperkalaemia the T waves become tall and peaked, while in hypokalaemia the T becomes lowered or inverted with an increase of the Q–T interval.

Heart block may be found in the severely ill child in all degrees. The E.C.G. picture varies from a prolongation of the P–R interval to a complete dissociation of atrial and ventricular events, ventricular complexes occurring far more infrequently than atrial. Complete heart block may cause a severe lowering of cardiac output.

Ventilation of a patient by mechanical means often causes E.C.G. changes particularly if large tidal volumes are being used. The alteration of the diameters of the chest caused by the positive pressure alters the position of the heart in the chest, which in turn alters the electrical axis of the heart. These changes are seen on the E.C.G. trace as a cyclical increase and decrease in the amplitude of the QRS complex.

Normality of the E.C.G. does not mean normality of the patient and the E.C.G. cannot be used in place of a pulse monitor. The E.C.G. does not give any indication of the haemodynamic changes occurring, nor does it indicate the strength of contraction of the heart. A triple purpose monitoring probe has been devised which may be placed in the oesophagus behind the heart. This probe has incorporated in it an E.C.G. electrode, an oesophageal stethoscope and a thermistor with which to measure temperature. This system may indeed be regarded as a life system sensor, for it is extremely unlikely, in the presence of a normal E.C.G., normal heart sounds and a normal temperature, that adequate blood flow would not be occurring. Interpretation of the E.C.G. must always be undertaken in conjunction with the clinical condition of the patient and can never be regarded as a substitute.

Tissue Perfusion

Blood flow through the tissues in adequate amount is required to support life. It is not possible as a routine to measure blood flow in the I.T.U. Ease of access is normally not available to the arterial blood supplies of major organs. Trauma inflicted on patients to insert monitoring probes to gain access to such vessels is to be deprecated as a routine procedure. Tissue flow is thus clinically assessed by inference. A pink warm periphery with a rapid capillary refill time can be taken to indicate adequate peripheral perfusion and *usually* adequacy of the deeper tissue perfusion, peripheral shut-down being one of the earliest signs of inadequacy of the circulation. The conscious level may be taken as a measure of the adequacy of cerebral perfusion, while normal E.C.G. and urinary output indicate normality of perfusion of the heart and kidneys. Individual aberrations of tissue perfusion are often difficult to assay clinically and it is the well-being of the whole that is taken as the indication of normality.

The Nervous System

The level of consciousness is best ascertained by clinical assessment and the conscious and unconscious patient are easy to differentiate. Unfortunately one rapidly becomes preoccupied with the 'in-between' states and the prognosis of these. The response of the older patient to spoken stimulus may be assessed and in the very young patients spontaneous movement or crying as a result of an auditory insult or a mild physical interference may well indicate that all is well. In the patient who does not respond to these mild stimuli or who does not show normal spontaneous activity, it becomes necessary to observe the pupillary response and size, the response to pain, the reflex responses and to estimate from these the depth or changing pattern of consciousness. It is not possible even after the most diligent examination to give short term prognostication as to the true progress or recoverability of the patient.

The electroencephalogram as a manifestation of the electrical activity of the brain would be thought to have a place as a monitor. Unfortunately, as a rapid dynamic measurement it is of little use, usually requiring an expert in this particular field to throw light on its significance. This problem is made worse in small children by the fact that the E.E.G. activity is undifferentiated and variable and of poor amplitude so that 'on the spot' assessment of the state of the brain by the E.E.G. is not usually possible.

Ventilation

Clinical assessment of ventilation is simple as one looks at the rate, the depth, the presence of distress and its degree, whether ventilation is noisy or not, and the patient's colour. This may seem adequate for the conscious, spontaneously breathing patient. Such clinical assessment is not sufficient in the case of a paralysed and ventilated patient who may have a good colour but in fact be underventilated. The collection of respired gases is much more difficult than it at first appears, and measurement of gas flow is particularly difficult in small children. The Wright respirometer is a useful instrument for adults but for small children has considerable errors. The ideal instrument to measure gas flow should have little effect on expiratory resistance and also on dead space. The pneumotachygraph may be used to calculate gas flow by measuring the pressure drop across a fine mesh screen placed across a tube, and the pressure drop will be proportional to the rate of flow. The principle is simple but the apparatus is difficult to use in practice since, for accurate measurement careful calibration is necessary, and the measurements must be made with the instrument at the same temperature as the gas which is being measured. At the present time the pneumotachygraph is not a suitable apparatus for continuous monitoring.

The apnoea monitor indicates whether the patient is breathing or not. Such a device is of particular importance in small children who are breathing spontaneously and are unattended for periods of time while in the I.T.U. The principle employed is simple. While some changing signal set up by spontaneous or controlled ventilation is received, the monitor is silent. If the signal stops for a predetermined period of time the monitor sounds and shows an alarm. A thermistor recording temperature changes in the gases close to the patient in a breathing circuit during inspiration and expiration will create a suitable signal. The impedance plethysmograph is probably better, as the electrodes are attached to either side of the patient's chest and changing electrical resistance between them is continuously measured. It must be remembered that this latter device is in reality monitoring chest movement and in the presence of obstruction there will be exaggerated chest movement but no ventilation.

It would appear that routine respiratory monitoring from the aspect of ventilation is still largely a clinical task; many instruments are devised to aid in this task but none can be relied upon absolutely in the role of continuous monitoring.

Temperature

Children, particularly very small infants, have far more difficulty in controlling body temperature than do adults. Their relatively small mass and large surface area make them far more subject to changes in the environment.

For continuous measurement of temperature the mercury and glass thermometer is at a disadvantage. Direct reading thermometry depends on the use of a thermocouple, heating which causes an electric current to pass whose voltage is proportional to the temperature and is constant for each degree of temperature change. This temperature can be displayed directly on the dial of an instrument which is in reality a device for measuring voltage. The resistance thermometer and the thermistor thermometer rely on change of resistance with temperature. The former has an increase in resistance in its sensing probe with the rise of temperature, while the latter has a fall; these changes can be measured and correlated to the change of temperature.

It must be decided where the monitoring probe should be applied to give a meaningful result. The temperature of the empty rectum is higher than other temperatures normally recorded while insulation by faeces renders rectal temperature recordings unreliable. The use of oesophageal and naso-pharyngeal sites is common and it is presumed that they give results representing the temperature of the brain stem, and of the mediastinum respectively. With temperature recording as with other monitoring the results obtained must be interpreted with caution and with clinical understanding of the situation.

Future development of monitoring would seem to lie with ever increasing miniaturisation of both the sensing and transduction devices and their ease of application, the removal of the read-out mechanisms from the patient to a remote site, the abandoning of wire connections and their replacement by radio transmission. Automation of monitoring would seem to be an obvious developmental trend together with the use of computerisation to set the limits of normality of any function, warning then being given as soon as abnormality occurs. This must also increase the complexity of the devices used. Such developments will give monitoring systems which will aid patient observation and elucidation of the problems to a degree better than is found at present, but they will never be able to supplant clinical observation, for this will be left when all else has failed.

CHAPTER 9

Ventilators

The practice of rhythmically inflating the lungs by artificial means has been found to be of great value in the treatment of respiratory failure, the causes of which are discussed elsewhere. Since it is not practical to do this by hand for any length of time, there are many machines which have been designed for the purpose.

It is not proposed to discuss those machines which exert negative pressure externally on the chest, as they are not much used these days. Only intermittent positive pressure machines will be described. The enormous number of such machines available indicates that there are few which suit every possible purpose. There are even fewer which are satisfactory for the special problems presented by infants.

CHOICE OF A VENTILATOR

A ventilator for a paediatric intensive care unit must be able efficiently to ventilate any patient from birth to adult size, and must be able to work equally well in the presence of normal lungs or highly abnormal ones. Humidification is essential, but apparatus dead space must be kept to a minimum. The dead space in some humidifiers is far too large for use with infants. It must also be remembered that water overload in infants is a real hazard. Accurate control of inspired oxygen concentration is important, because there is evidence to suggest that high oxygen concentrations, combined with pressure on the lungs may contribute to death from 'ventilator lung'—(a condition characterised by decreasing compliance of the lungs, increasing opacity on X-ray, associated with small translucent areas, and an 'air bronchogram': microscopy shows hyaline membranes in the alveoli).

Since intensive care units tend to be places of stress for both patients and nursing staff, it is helpful if a ventilator is fairly quiet in operation—on the other hand, an alteration in noise may serve as an alarm to warn of machine failure. Ease of sterilisation is important, as patients on ventilators are very susceptible to infection.

To summarise, some desirable features of a ventilator for use in this type of unit are:
1. Ability accurately to deliver a tidal volume of 15 ml to 1000 ml.
2. Ability to deliver this volume against high resistance and/or low compliance.
3. Ability to deliver low flow rates.
4. Rate control from 15/minute to 40/minute.
5. Accurate control of inspired oxygen concentration.
6. A variable inspiratory: expiratory ratio (I:E ratio).
7. Good humidification for all tidal volumes.
8. Ease of sterilisation.
9. Quietness of operation.
10. Ability to apply a variable expiratory resistance.

The type or types of machine chosen for an individual unit depend on personal preference and also on the conditions treated. Some units may prefer to have all of one type—this certainly ensures that everyone becomes familiar with its operation. It is probably preferable to have two or three different types, to cope with various problems. A greater variety could become unwieldy.

MONITORING OF VENTILATION

It is essential to have some method of ensuring adequate ventilation of the patient at all times. For this purpose, several devices are used. Most machines incorporate a pressure manometer which reads airway pressure at the mouth, or at the machine, and this being connected to the patient by a wide-bore tubing of low resistance. Due to resistance in the airways, the pressure in the alveoli may be very different from that at the mouth. Many machines have a blow-off valve, preset at, say, 70 mm Hg, to protect the lungs from excessive pressure. Observations of fluctuations of the pressure reading on the dial will give an indication of altering compliance and resistance if the machine is volume-cycled.

Measurement of expired tidal volume is important. This is easily done by meters like the Wright respirometer, but these do not read accurately below a minute volume of four litres. Since the normal minute volume of many children is less than this, measurement of their tidal volumes is difficult. It can be done with a pneumotachygraph which derives gas flow rate from the difference in pressures measured on each side of a large orifice in the circuit. Such apparatus is bulky and expensive.

Adequacy of ventilation is usually measured by blood gas studies, chiefly the P_{CO_2}. It is not advisable to keep this too low, as vasoconstriction occurs, especially important in cerebral vessels. On the other hand, hypercarbia leads to central nervous system depression, and increased cardiac irritability.

PHYSIOLOGY OF ARTIFICIAL VENTILATION

Gas exchange in the lungs can be maintained efficiently by artificial ventilation, but the pressures produced in the thorax are quite different from those in normal respiration, and there are some potentially harmful effects.

In normal breathing, inspiration is initiated by an upward and outward movement of the lower ribs, and by descent of the diaphragm, thus increasing the internal capacity of the chest, and causing a lower pressure in the alveoli than at the mouth. This pressure can be measured by a balloon in the oesophagus. Air is sucked into the lungs.

Expiration is effected by relaxation of the muscles, a passive return of the chest wall to its original position, and a return of alveolar pressure towards atmospheric. Since the heart and great vessels are inside the thorax, the suction effect during inspiration assists the flow of blood into them from peripheral veins.

If a mechanical ventilator is used, the intrathoracic pressure changes are reversed. Positive pressure from the machine drives gas into the lungs via the airway, and alveolar pressure rises above atmospheric, which interferes with return of blood to the heart. During expiration the chest wall returns to its resting position, and the alveolar pressure falls to atmospheric. During this time, blood can return to the heart. If the patient has a normal cardiovascular system, compensation occurs by a rise of venous pressure so that sufficient blood reaches the heart and the cardiac output is not reduced. However, if the circulating blood volume is low, compensation may be inadequate. The length of time during which positive pressure is applied to the lungs should be as short as possible, but it must be long enough for an adequate volume of gas to enter the lungs. That is to say, the mean intrathoracic pressure should be kept as low as practicable. (This takes into account pressures reached during inspiration and expiration, and depends on the wave-form delivered by the ventilator). The exception to this rule is in the presence of pulmonary oedema, which may be greatly improved by keeping the mean intrathoracic pressure high. To keep the mean pressure low, suction may be applied to the airway during expiration. This causes some danger of collapse of abnormal airways, and can hinder expiration in the presence of emphysema.

A further potential hazard of positive-pressure respiration is rupture of the lungs, due to high pressure being exerted on the alveoli. This can be minimised by careful setting of the machine and usually only occurs when the lung has weakened areas, e.g. emphysema, or areas of uneven compliance, so that high pressures needed to inflate the stiff areas may rupture the more normal areas. If the patient is breathing against the ventilator, very high pressure can be created, and rupture may occur. When it does, it is usually interstitial, and air tracks along vessels to the mediastinum. From there it may rupture into the pleura and cause a pneumothorax.

MODE OF ACTION OF VENTILATORS

The action of a ventilator can be divided into four phases:
 1. Inspiratory phase
 2. Change-over from inspiration to expiration
 3. Expiratory phase
 4. Change over from expiration to inspiration.

The following account is simplified and those interested must refer to larger reference books.

1. The Inspiratory Phase

This phase must deliver a gas mixture to the patient, and the

Ventilators

patterns of gas flow, volume, and pressure produced in the lungs depend on the characteristics of the ventilator and on the condition of the lungs.

There are basically two types of ventilator—flow generators and pressure generators.

In the former type the ventilator determines the pattern of flow into the lungs and the volume delivered and the resultant pressure depend on the characteristics of the lungs.

In the latter type the ventilator determines the pressure pattern, and the resultant flow and volume patterns depend on the characteristics of the lungs.

Flow generators

(a) *constant flow generators:* These produce a steady rise in alveolar pressure and volume until the end of inspiration, the magnitude depending on the flow rate. Examples are Blease, Bird (without air mix) and the Amsterdam infant ventilator. The latter two are driven by gas pipeline pressure; the former is a mechanical volume pump.

(b) *non-constant flow generators* (sine-wave generators): The flow rises to a maximum about the middle of inspiration and declines towards the end. Examples are the Cape, Starling pump and Engström. These machines act by driving a piston or concertina bag by a mechanical linkage from a constant speed motor.

Pressure generators

(a) *constant pressure generators:* Pressure may be produced by the action of a weight (variable, depending on magnitude of pressure desired), acting on a concertina bag, as in the East-Radcliffe. Alternatively, pressure may be produced by an injector operated by gas from a pipeline, e.g. Bird (on air mix setting). The resultant pressure is always less than the pipeline pressure and depends on the flow-rate control setting.

The action of an injector depends on gas at a high pressure being driven through a small hole. The gas jet enters a larger chamber open to the gas to be entrained (in this case air). The force of the jet draws air into the chamber, causing a mixed gas to pass out and act as the driving gas.

(b) *non-constant pressure generators*: One example of this type is the Barnet, which has a concertina bag compressed by a spring. As the bag empties, the spring relaxes and the pressure exerted on the bag decreases.

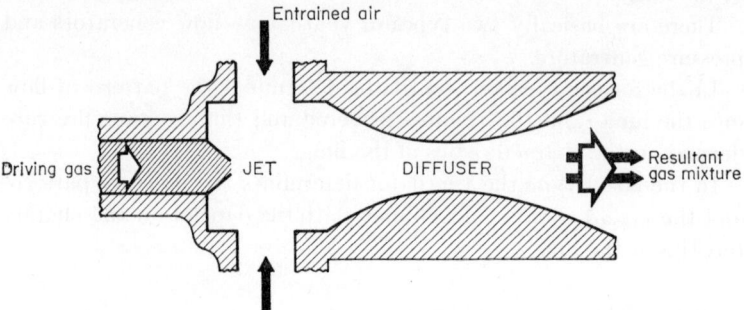

FIG. 9.1 Diagram of gas injector.

2. Cycling at the end of inspiration

No matter how inspiration is produced, it must be terminated. During inspiration, time is elapsing, pressure is building to a peak, flow of gas is occurring and the volume delivered is increasing.

Inspiration is terminated when one or several of these factors has reached a predetermined value.

Therefore the ventilator may have:
 (a) time cycling
 (b) volume cycling
 (c) pressure cycling
 (d) a mixture of several of these.

Time cycling

The length of time from beginning to end of inspiration is controlled by a timing device, and is independent of lung characteristics. The device may be electronic (e.g. Barnet), electro-mechanical (e.g. East-Radcliffe) or pneumatic (e.g. Air Shields). The volume delivered to the patient, and the pressure produced, depend on the inspiratory phase and on lung characteristics.

Volume cycling

The volume is preset on a piston or concertina bag, and the length of inspiration, and the pressure produced in the lungs, depend on the characteristics of the latter. If there is any leak in the circuit the

Ventilators

whole volume will not be delivered to the patient, and this can be noticed if a watch is kept on airway pressure and expired volume.

Pressure cycling

The preset pressure at which inspiration is to cease is measured at the mouth or at the machine. Cycling occurs without reference to the time taken to reach this pressure or the volume of gas delivered to the patient, both of which depend on lung characteristics. The pressure is usually sensed by a diaphragm which moves as pressure rises and operates electrical contacts (Barnet) or a spring-loaded mechanical trip (Blease), or overcomes the attraction of a magnet for an iron plate (Bird).

If there is a leak in the circuit, the cycling pressure may never be reached—i.e., inspiration becomes infinite. This can be quickly noticed.

Mixed cycling

A ventilator (e.g. Barnet Mk III) may have two or more possible types of cycling, and the type is selected to suit the patient. Most volume-cycled ventilators are also time-cycled.

3. The Expiratory Phase

In most cases expiration is effected by connecting the patient's airway to the atmosphere, a valve being opened either near the patient or in the machine. In the latter case the circuit must be one-way—i.e. have two tubes, one for inspiration and one for expiration, connected by a Y junction, otherwise considerable rebreathing would occur. Gas will flow from the higher pressure in the lungs to atmosphere until the pressures are equal, given time.

In a few special circumstances it may be required to assist expiration by suction, or to retard it by an expiratory resistance. The latter may be simply a clamp across the expiratory hose, a cap placed over the expiratory port (e.g. Bird) or spring loading of the expiratory valve.

4. Changeover from expiration to inspiration

The cycling mechanisms may be the same as those used at the end of inspiration, although the same mechanism is not necessarily used for both in the same machine. There is an additional method which may be used—patient triggering.

(a) *time cycling:* By far the commonest mechanism.

(b) *volume cycling:* This can only be used if expiration is assisted.

(c) *pressure cycling:* The end of expiration occurs when a preset pressure at the mouth is reached. This may be a method of keeping a positive pressure exerted on the airway (i.e. positive-positive ventilation).

(d) *patient cycling or triggering:* Inspiration is initiated by patient effort which produces a negative pressure in the circuit. This is usually sensed by a diaphragm, the movement of which initiates the inspiratory phase. Usually the machine has some other triggering device in case patient effort fails. Patient triggering has little to recommend it in infants.

PRACTICAL POINTS IN THE MANAGEMENT OF VENTILATION IN CHILDREN

The problem faced in ventilating small patients is that a small but accurate volume must be delivered against the high resistance provided by narrow tubes, and against lungs which often have poor compliance. It is a help if the machine can deliver very low flow rates. If it cannot do this then it may need to be modified. Several methods are available:

(a) reduce inflating flow by either

(i) place a resistance in series with the ventilator, i.e. a screw clamp across the inspiratory hose.

or

(ii) modify the ventilator.

(b) dispose of excess flow by either

(i) a leak in the circuit.

or

(ii) a device in parallel to absorb the excess flow—usually the ventilator inflates both the patient and a dummy lung. The compliance of the dummy lung must be carefully adjusted.

Although one of these methods may be used if necessary, it is far better to use a ventilator specially designed for infants.

Most ventilators can be made to accomplish inspiration. It is the cycling mechanism at the end of inspiration that is important.

Ventilators

Pressure cycling

If there is a kink in the tubing or some other obstruction to inspiration, the machine will cycle very rapidly, and very small volumes will be delivered. This can easily be recognised and the trouble set right if possible. However, if the cause is airways obstruction or lungs of poor compliance, then the inspiratory flow rate must be slowed to allow more time before the cycling pressure is reached. It may not be able to be slowed enough. If such a machine is being used to ventilate a patient in whom the airways resistance suddenly falls (e.g. asthma) or the lung compliance suddenly increases (e.g. pulmonary oedema), a much larger volume will be delivered to the patient before the cycling pressure is reached. This may be harmful if not quickly noticed.

Volume cycling

If airway resistance is high or lung compliance low, delivery of a set volume will result in high pressures at the mouth which do not necessarily reflect those in the lungs. However, if conditions improve suddenly, all that will happen is that the pressure at the mouth will fall. Severe hyperventilation will not result. However, if a leak develops in the circuit it may not be noticed at once.

The dead space of humidifiers must be watched with small children, also the dead space of elephant tubing and patient connections. It is better to use narrow non-expansile tubing, and one-way circuits.

Suitable tidal and minute volumes may be estimated from prepared nomograms, or from highly inaccurate formulae. Adequacy of ventilation is gauged by P_aCO_2. Rapid ventilation rates are unnecessary in children, and may indeed be harmful. Sufficient time must be given to provide even distribution of gas in the lungs and for gas exchange to take place.

The inspired oxygen concentration should always be as low as possible to be compatible with physiological requirements. Estimation of blood P_aO_2 is very useful but obtaining arterial blood can be difficult in babies.

If possible ventilator tubing should be changed frequently to discourage infection, and water should not be allowed to stand for long periods of time because it provides a good culture medium for bacteria.

The general nutritional state and hydration of the patient must of course always be attended to meticulously.

HUMIDIFICATION

Artificial ventilation of the lungs for a prolonged period necessitates the introduction of an artificial airway, whether it be an endotracheal tube or a tracheostomy. In either case, the nose is bypassed. The normal function of the nose is to heat air to about 35°C and to add water vapour to it. Water content in the trachea is normally about 35 mg/litre (air fully saturated with water at body temperature contains 44 mg/litre). Warm moist air is essential to keep bronchial secretions liquid, and for correct functioning of the ciliated respiratory mucosa. These cilia beat in unison and assist in driving mucus towards the larynx, but in cold, dry conditions they stop working, mucus dries, and becomes sticky. The only means of removing this mucus is then by coughing or suction, and it may cause obstruction of the bronchi.

Too much water delivered to the lungs will result in over-hydration of the patient and patchy lung collapse.

Ideally the air delivered via an artificial airway should be at a temperature of 30 to 36°C and a humidity of 30 to 40 mg/litre.

There are ways of aiming to achieve one or both of these ideals, but none is entirely satisfactory.

Water is usually used, but saline may be preferred.

Humidifiers are normally situated in the inspiratory line to the patient. Some are in the gas feed line to the ventilator (e.g. Loosco).

Types of Humidifiers

Artificial nose

This consists of a wire mesh disc situated in the catheter mount to the patient. Expired gases pass back through the mesh, which is warmed and retains some water. Both warmth and moisture are transmitted to the inspired gas on the next inspiration. This type of humidifier is only moderately efficient, and does tend to increase resistance to respiration, which is a bad thing in children. Blockage readily occurs if a mucous plug is coughed up, and this may be dangerous.

Instillation of water or saline

Amounts of 1 to 5 ml may be instilled into the airway at intervals from $\frac{1}{4}$ to 1 hour. Some humidity is produced but it is intermittent and not very efficient. It is an effective way of loosening dried plugs of mucus, however.

Ventilators

Infusion from a drip set may be used, into the inspiratory tube close to the patient. Humidity so produced is far from ideal, and there is a danger of drowning the patient unless the rate is very accurately controlled.

Nebulisers

(a) *gas-driven:* These work on the 'scent spray' principle, and are used on gas-driven pressure-cycled machines such as the Bird and Bennett.

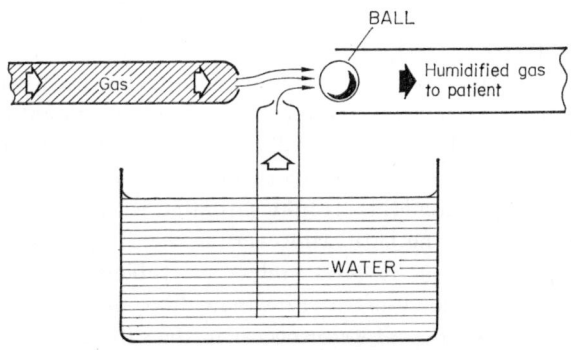

FIG. 9.2 Diagram of gas-driven nebuliser.

Compressed gas emerges from a fine hole and blows over the top of a narrow tube, the other end of which dips into water. The force of the gas jet draws water up the tube and breaks it into droplets. The largest of these are collected on a plastic ball, and the rest pass with the gas along the tube to the patient.

Such a nebuliser is capable of delivering humidity of up to 29 mg/litre if unheated, and 50 mg/litre if heated.

The disadvantages are that much condensation takes place in the tubing, causing some obstruction. Moreover bacteria are readily carried by droplets and may be transmitted directly to the patient. Water should, therefore, be sterile before use and should not be allowed to stand for long periods. Ventilator tubing should be changed frequently.

(b) *ultrasonic:* Water or saline is dropped on a disc which is vibrated at ultrasonic speeds. The water is broken up into a very fine mist of droplets, which pass along to the patient with the inspired gas. These droplets are so fine that they do not condense in the tubing, and they pass readily into the smaller air passages of the lungs (and even out again). They are also very well suited to carrying bacteria.

These nebulisers are so efficient that it is very easy to over-hydrate a patient, and special care is needed if they are used with children.

Nebulisers may also be used to administer drugs, such as mucolytic substances, bronchodilators, hydrocortisone and muscle relaxants.

Water-bath Humidifiers

These must be heated to be of any use, and there are two types—the draw-over type, in which gas is drawn over the surface of the water, picking up water vapour, and the bubble-through type, where gas is bubbled through the heated water, to increase the amount of water vapour picked up. It is then normally passed through a water trap to allow condensation of excessive moisture.

Gas leaving the humidifier is fully saturated with water vapour at the temperature of the bath. However, as the gas passes along the tubing to the patient, it cools, unless the tubing is insulated, or 'lagged', and the amount of water it can hold is considerably reduced. Therefore condensation of water occurs in the tubing.

Precautions must be taken to ensure that the water does not overheat, otherwise the patient's airway may be scalded.

Water vapour, as opposed to droplets, does not carry bacteria, so contamination is not so likely. However, tubing should be changed regularly as the water accumulating in it will provide a culture medium.

A BRIEF DESCRIPTION OF SOME VENTILATORS SUITABLE FOR USE IN A PAEDIATRIC INTENSIVE THERAPY UNIT

Amsterdam Infant Ventilator (Loosco)

This ventilator operates as a constant flow generator from gas flowmeters during inspiration. Both the changeover at the end of inspiration and that at the end of expiration are time cycled, by an electronic timer operating a solenoid valve. Expiration may be retarded or assisted, by varying the amount of gas flowing through an

Ventilators

injector. The I:E ratio may be adjusted from 1:1 to 1:3 and rates from 20 to 55/minute.

The humidifier is a heated bubble-through type with a water trap, situated before the ventilator.

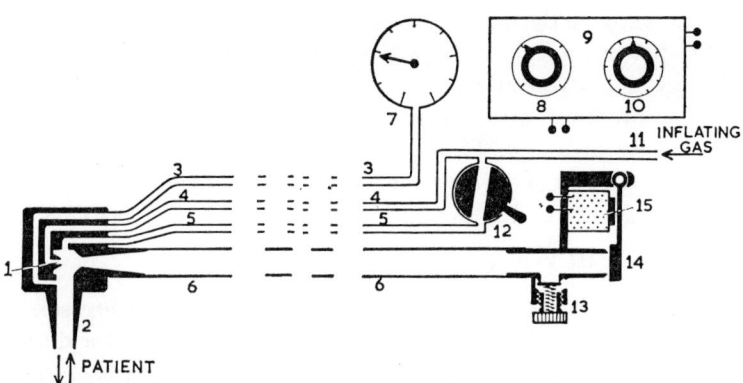

1. Injector
2. Endotracheal-tube connexion
3. Manometer tube
4. Supply tube to injector
5. Supply tube to airway
6. Expiratory tube
7. Manometer
8. 'Inspiration % of cycle'
9. Timing control unit
10. 'Respiratory frequency' control
11. Inflating-gas inlet
12. Negative-pressure control tap
13. Safety-valve
14. Expiratory valve
15. Solenoid

FIG. 9.3 Diagram of the 'Amsterdam Infant Ventilator' (by courtesy of Prof. W. W. Mushin).

On one side of the ventilator there is a chart which indicates the relationship between the gas flow (as set, as a mixture of air and oxygen on the flowmeters), the length of the inspiratory phase (determined by setting the ventilation rate and the I:E ratio), and the resultant tidal volume. By estimating the required tidal volume, one can set the machine for use. In practice the flow rate may have to be increased, due to losses from leaks around uncuffed endotracheal tubes.

Gas flows continuously through the humidifier and the machine and along the inspiratory flow line to the patient. During inspiration, the expiratory valve is held closed electronically, and the gas flow directed into the patient's lungs. Resultant pressure at the mouth is read on the manometer. At the end of inspiration the expiratory valve is allowed to open and the fresh gas flows along the expiratory tube, together with the expired gases from the patient. If a negative pressure is required during expiration, some of the fresh gas flow is directed through the injector exerting suction on the airway. If no gas is directed through the injector the pressure at the end of expiration is always slightly positive.

The ventilator is fitted with a blow-off valve to prevent generation of excessive pressures. There is also a device for manual control of gas flow. This is a useful machine for ventilating infants.

Barnet Mark III Ventilator

This machine is very complicated and this account is necessarily simplified. It functions as a non-constant pressure generator during inspiration, due to the action of a spring on a concertina bag. Fresh gas enters this bag from flow meters and the oxygen concentration may be controlled. Cycling at the end of inspiration may be either by time, volume, or pressure and each mode has its own set of controls, marked in colours. The expiratory phase may be to atmospheric or a negative pressure but if a positive pressure is required, a clamp must be placed across the expiratory hose. There is a patient-triggering device, and pressure at the mouth may be read on a manometer.

The patient circuit of most use in prolonged ventilation is a non-rebreathing, or 'open' one. As supplied this consists of wide-bore elephant tubing, the expansile nature of which may lead to errors if used with small children. Rigid narrower plastic tubing may be used instead.

Gases are usually humidified by a heated water draw-over type in the inspiratory line. The large dead space in this may also lead to errors in small children.

Expired tidal volumes in larger children and adults may be read from a Wright respirometer incorporated in the machine. At smaller minute volumes this is not accurate. However, the machine, with the open circuit, is a 'minute volume divider'—the minute volume is set on the gas flow meters and the tidal volume depends on the rate setting, provided there are no leaks in the circuit. In any case, ventilation should be monitored by blood gas estimations.

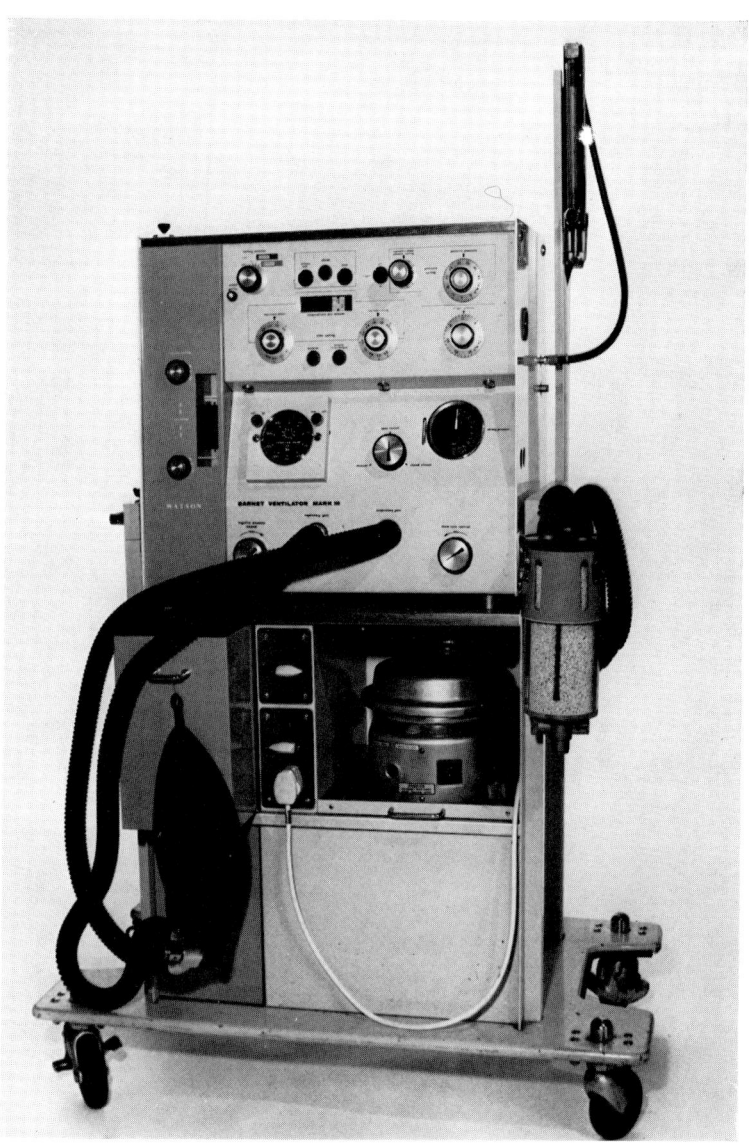

Fig. 9.4 Barnet Mk III Ventilator.

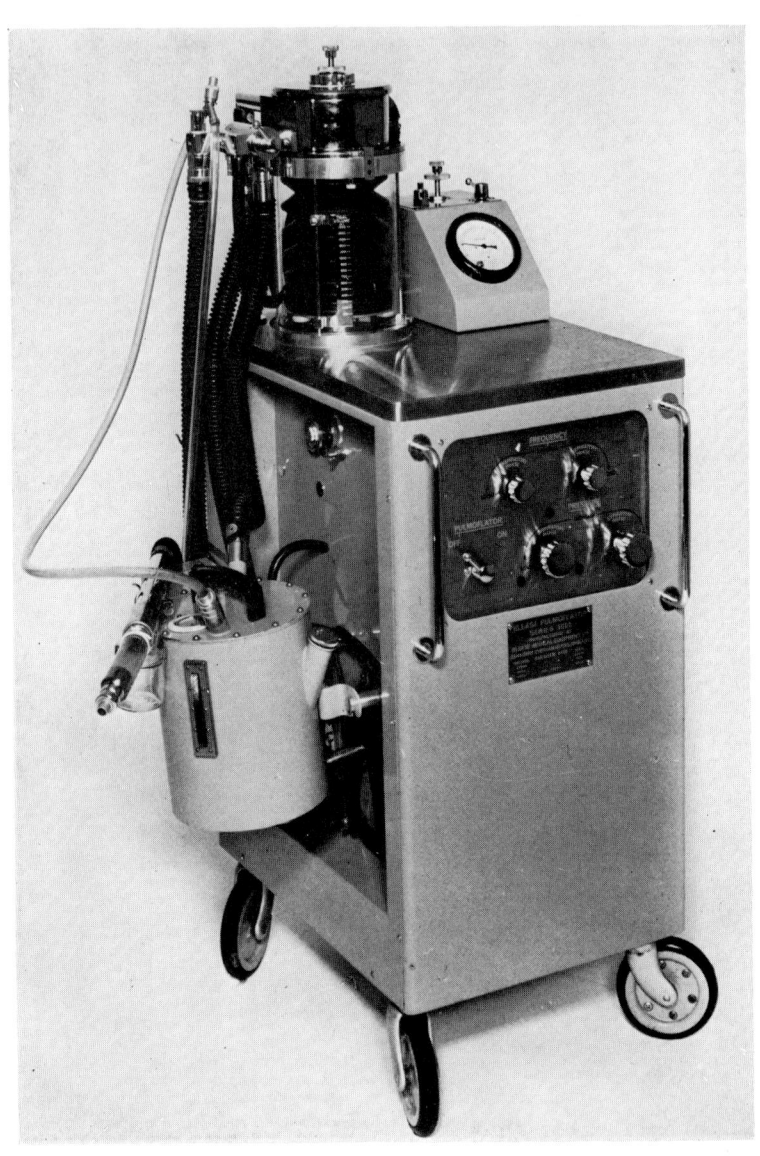

FIG. 9.6 Blease pulmoflator series 5000.

Ventilators

Bird Mark 7 and 8

The Mk. 7 is the basic design. The Mk. 8 has the addition of a negative pressure applicable during the expiratory phase, and uses a different valve assembly incorporating an injector. During the inspiratory phase, without air mix, the machine functions as a flow generator. With the air-mix control pulled out, the patient is inflated by an injector and the machine functions as a pressure generator. These different modes of operation have practical significance regarding efficiency of ventilation, apart from the differences in inspired oxygen concentration.

Changeover from inspiration to expiration is pressure cycled. Expiration is to atmospheric pressure, but negative pressure may be applied with the Mk. 8. The end of expiration is normally time-cycled but may be patient triggered.

The pressure reached in the machine is measured on the manometer. Humidification is by cold-water nebulisation. Tidal volume cannot be read from the machine. In larger patients it can be read from a respirometer attached to the expiratory valve port. A cap may be fitted over this port to retard expiration.

The ventilator consists of a box, divided into two compartments by a central column which houses various gas flow pathways. The left hand compartment is open to the atmosphere, and the right hand compartment is a pressure chamber in direct communication with the patient's airway via a wide-bore tube. The pressure compartment extends through a hole in the central column behind a diaphragm on the atmospheric side. A ceramic spindle is free to move across the hole in the central column, and it is so grooved that when it moves to the right, gas can flow from the pipeline into the pressure chamber and so to the patient, but when it moves to the left the gas flow is cut off. Attached to either end of this spindle are two soft iron plates, so that movement of the plates causes movement of the spindle. Movement is caused by the alternate attraction for each plate by two magnets, one in each compartment. These magnets can be moved by a screw, to alter the force of attraction for each plate.

At the end of inspiration the spindle is over to the left and the left hand plate is attracted to its magnet. Inspiration is initiated by a lever which pushes the plate away from the magnet. This causes the right hand plate to be attracted by its magnet, and gas flows past the

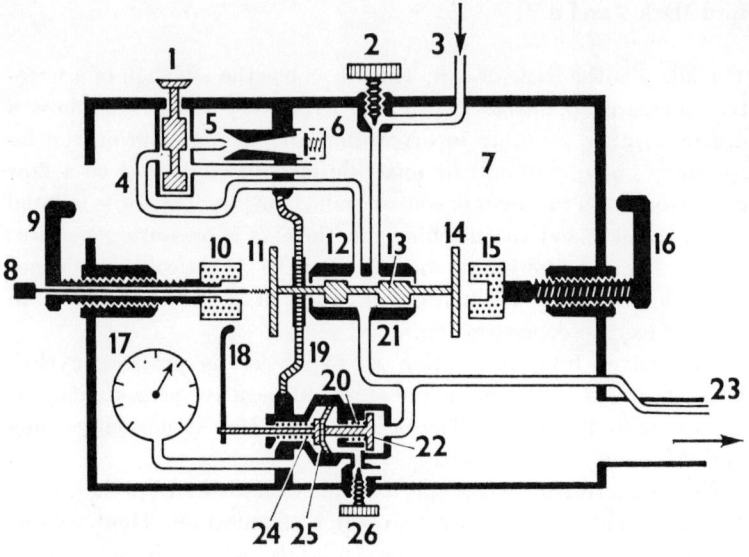
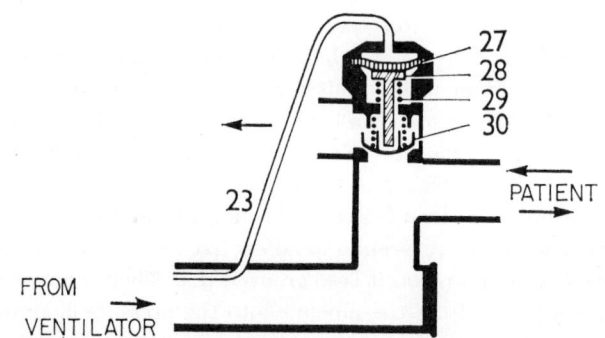

FIG. 9.5 Diagrams of the Bird Mark 7 Ventilator and expiratory valve assembly (by courtesy of Prof. W. W. Mushin).

1. 'Air-mix' control
2. 'Inspiratory time flowrate' control
3. Driving-gas inlet
4. Connecting tube
5. Injector
6. One-way valve
7. Main chamber
8. Manual-cycling control
9. 'Sensitivity effort' control
10. Magnet
11. Soft-iron plate
12. Outlet
13. Ceramic sliding valve
14. Soft-iron plate
15. Magnet
16. 'Inspiratory pressure limit' control

Ventilators

spindle into the pressure compartment. As more gas is delivered to the patient the airway pressure rises, and also causes the diaphragm to bulge out to the left. Eventually it bulges so far that the left hand plate is attracted to its magnet, breaking the attraction of the right hand pair. The force required to do this depends on the proximity of the right hand magnet to the plate, and this is preset as a cycling pressure. As the spindle moves to the left, the gas flow is cut off, and expiration occurs. During inspiration the expiratory valve has been kept shut by gas flow down a narrow tube to the diaphragm in the valve. This flow stops during expiration and the valve opens freely.

The cycle keeps repeating itself. If the left hand magnet is far away from its plate (i.e. the sensitivity setting is low) then an inspiratory effort by the patient will be sufficient to move the diaphragm in the machine, pull the left hand plate off the magnet, and initiate inspiration.

If the air mix control is pulled out, the inspiratory gas flows through an injector in the left hand chamber, entraining air to mix with the driving oxygen.

Theoretically this should provide the patient with an inspired oxygen concentration of 40 per cent. However, the nebulizer is driven by 100 per cent oxygen, and the measured oxygen delivered to the patient may be anything from 60 to 90 per cent. The efficiency of the injector also depends partly on the rate of gas flow, which may need to be very low to ventilate babies. The length of inspiration may be increased by decreasing the flow rate, and decreased by increasing the flow rate, for a certain pressure setting, thereby altering the I:E ratio.

For use with children, the adult circuit must be modified as its dead space is too large. This is accomplished by use of a 'Q' circuit, which consists of a Y junction, at the patient end. One tube is the inspiratory line from the machine, the other, the expiratory line to the expiratory valve. If a Mk. 8 is used, expiration may be assisted by suction.

---

17. Manometer
18. Striking arm
19. Diaphragm
20. Spring
21. Outlet
22. Piston
23. Small-bore tube
24. Spring
25. Diaphragm
26. 'Expiratory time' control
27. Diaphragm
28. Push rod
29. Spring
30. Expiratory valve

In an attempt to have a more variable inspired oxygen concentration, combined with the possibility of fast rates of ventilation, the infant J circuit has been devised. The ventilator is driven by compressed air, and a controlled flow of oxygen is added to the humidifier during inspiration. The circuit is one-way, but the expiratory valve is very light, and worked by a system of injectors.

To set up the ventilator for use, one selects the driving gas and circuit suitable, and adjusts the sensitivity setting, flow rate control, and pressure limit all to an arbitrary figure of 15. The machine is connected to the patient and the controls readjusted as necessary, to obtain the desired ventilation. The rate is set by unscrewing the 'expiratory time for APNEA' control.

Blease Pulmoflator Series 5000

This ventilator is a flow generator, and may be either pressure cycled, or time cycled and volume limited. If the set pressure is in excess of that required to deliver the required volume to the patient then the machine is volume limited, and the pressure is held for the length of inspiration.

The I:E ratio is readily variable, and there is a good range of frequency. Pressure at the mouth is read on a manometer. End-expiratory pressure may be varied from negative to positive, and patient triggering is possible.

The machine consists of an electrical air compressor, the flow from which is controlled in a complicated way, and then passes into a rigid plastic compartment to compress a concertina bag in order to deliver a volume from 200 to 1500 ml. This concertina bag is fed with a gas mixture from a reservoir bag. If this bag collapses during inspiration, air is entrained to the required volume. Using the open circuit, as the concertina bag is compressed gas passes along one hose, through a heated water, draw-over type humidifier, to the patient, and during expiration through the other hose to a one-way valve on the machine.

For infants, a paediatric circuit must be substituted for the open circuit. It consists of a small rebreathing bag attached to a one-way circuit of rigid plastic tubes. If the desired minute volume is fed into this bag, which is completely collapsed at each inspiration, then the machine acts as a minute volume divider. No humidifier is supplied for this circuit.

Ventilators

Bourns Paediatric Ventilator

Especially designed to ventilate neonates, this machine has an electric motor, which drives a piston to inflate the patient with a selected gas mixture. The valves are operated by a solenoid. It is a constant flow generator, both volume and time cycled.

Maximum tidal volume is 50 ml, and frequency may be varied from 20 to 110/minute. No negative pressure may be applied during expiration.

Engström Ventilator

This ventilator has a very complicated mechanism. Basically, a piston, driven by an electric motor, is used to compress a reservoir bag, containing the gas mixture to be delivered to the patient. This is done through a one-way circuit. Provided the reservoir bag is completely collapsed with each inspiration the machine is a minute volume divider. Air is drawn into the bag according to a 'closing valve' setting and oxygen can be added from a flow meter, the total minute volume being the sum of the two. Expired volume may be monitored with a respirometer.

During the inspiratory phase the ventilator acts as an increasing pressure generator and is time cycled. I:E ratio is usually 1:2. A pressure limit can be set for inspiration, and any excess gas is disposed of through a water manometer. Expiration may be retarded or a negative pressure applied. A heated water humidifier is supplied.

A nomogram for calculation of the required minute volume from the size of the patient is provided. For infants the wide elephant tubing should be replaced with rigid plastic tubing.

Starling Pump

This is a very simple ventilator, originally designed for animals, and a modified version can be used to ventilate infants.

Three sizes are available, to deliver maximum tidal volumes of 250, 500 and 800 ml respectively.

An electric motor drives a piston which supplies the patient with atmospheric air, or with a gas mixture. Expiration occurs through a valve on the machine.

The rate can be varied from 14 to 45 per minute and the I:E ratio is fixed at 1:2.

The machine acts as a non-constant (sine-wave) flow generator and is both volume and time cycled. Expiration is to atmospheric pressure only. No humidifier is supplied.

FURTHER READING

MUSHIN, W. W. *et al*. *Automatic ventilation of the lungs*, 2nd edition. (Blackwell) 1969.

ROBINSON, J. S. 'Choice of a Ventilator' in *Modern Trends in Anaesthesia* 3. (Butterworth) 1966.

CHAMNEY, ANNE 'Humidification requirements and techniques', *Anaesthesia* Vol. **24,** p. 602. 1969.

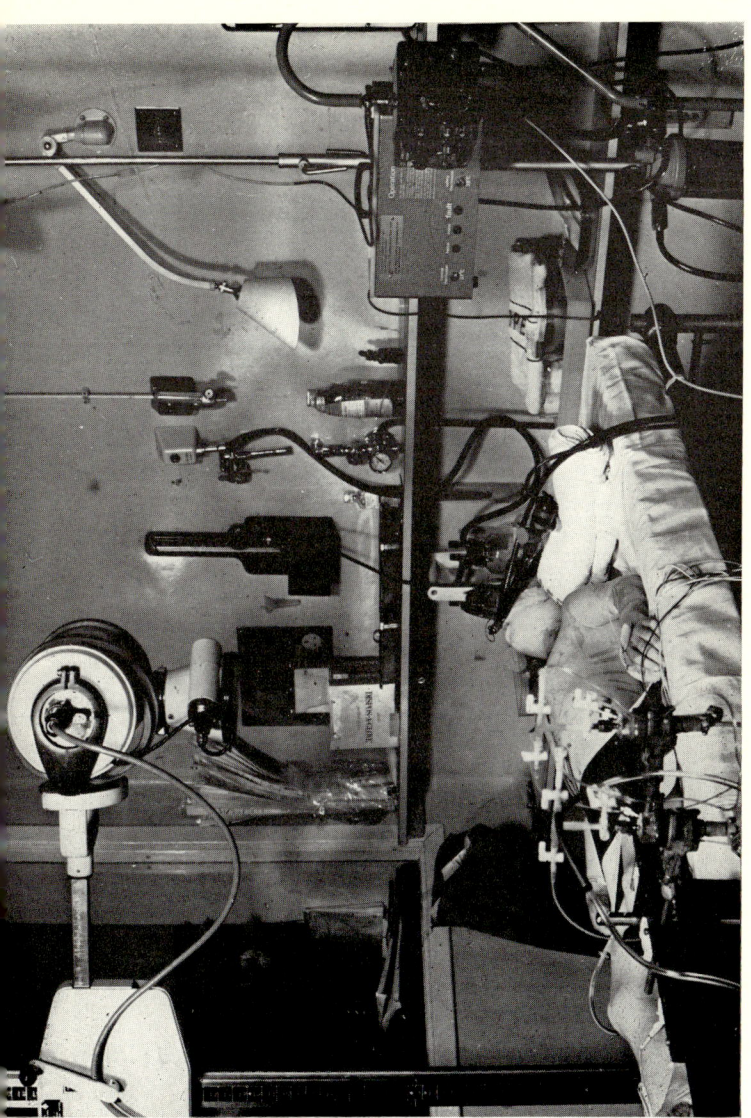

FIG. 10.1 A chest radiograph is taken with the mobile X-ray set immediately after a cardiac operation. The film cassette has been placed underneath the chest.

facing p. 124

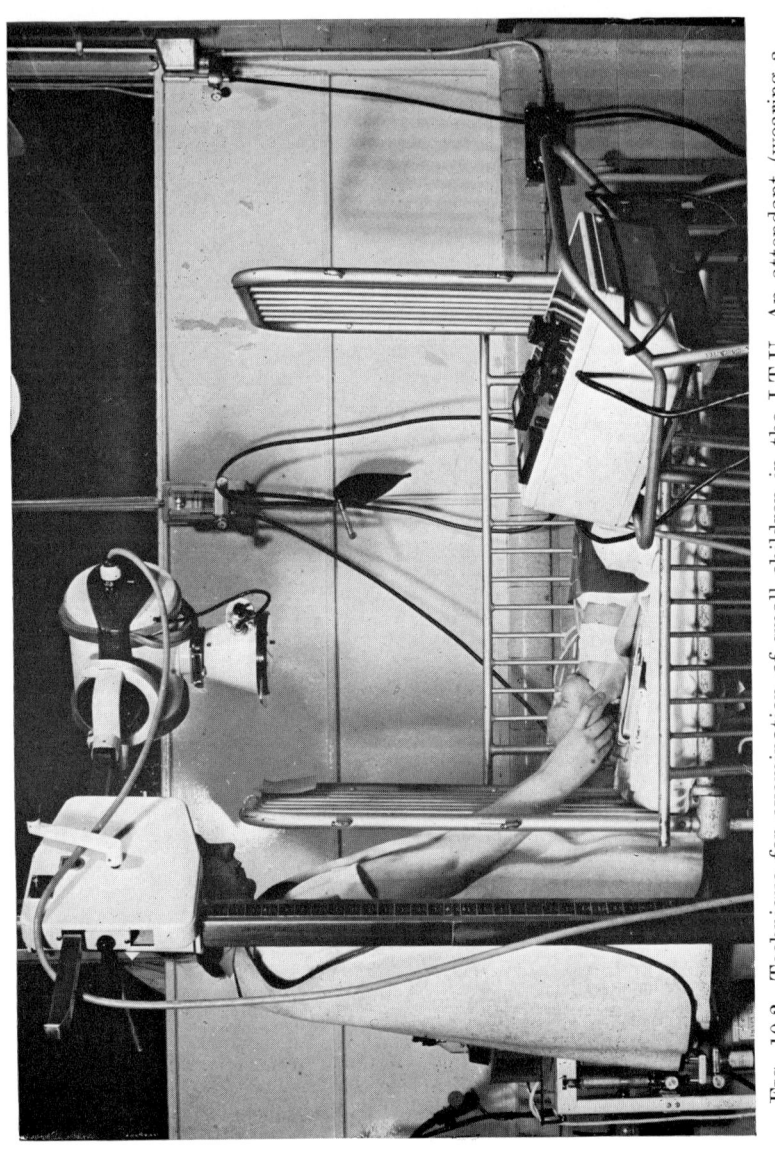

FIG. 10.2 Technique for examination of small children in the I.T.U. An attendant (wearing a protective apron) held the child's extended arms alongside the head, keeping the chest straight.

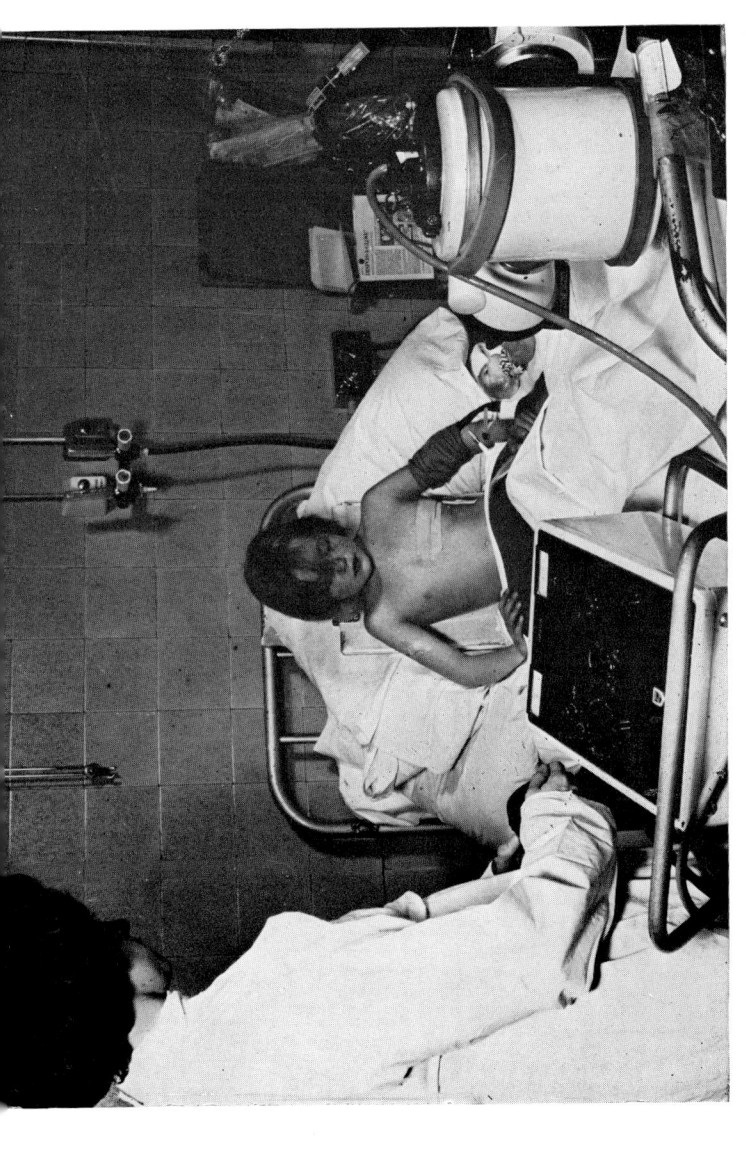

FIG. 10.3 A chest film is taken a few days after operation. The child is well enough to sit up and co-operate. In this case the direction of the X-ray beam is horizontal.

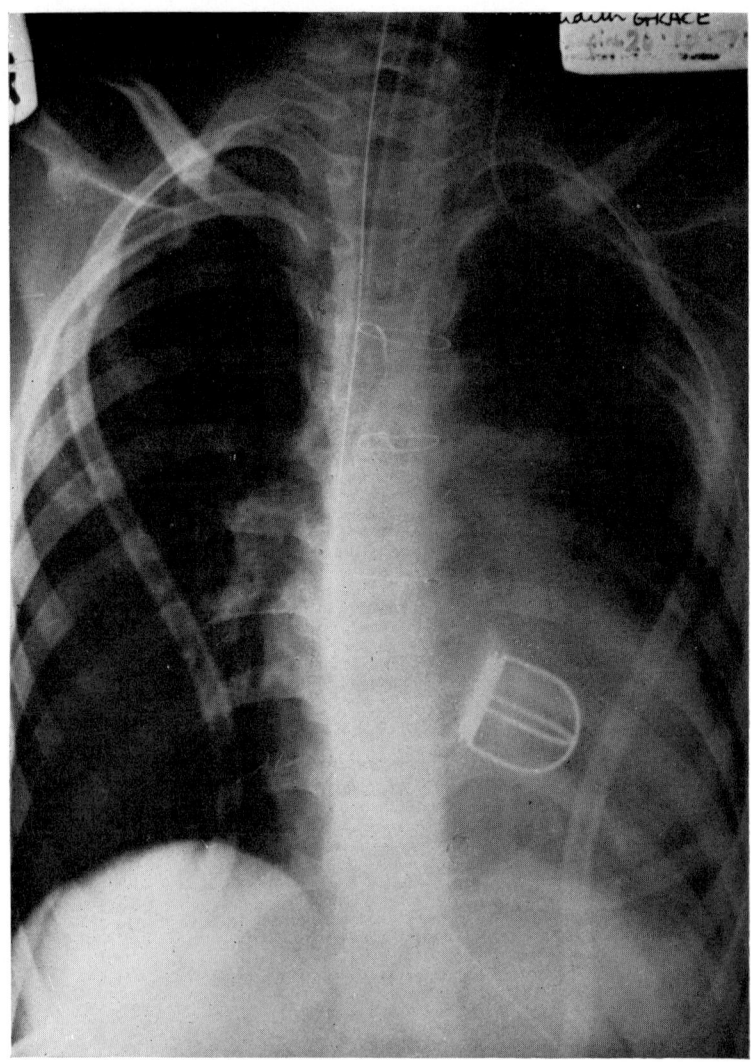

Fig. 10.4 A postoperative chest film showing intercostal drainage tubes, an endotracheal tube, a tube for aspirating the stomach and a venous catheter. Their position should be observed when viewing the radiograph. (The mitral valve has been replaced by a prosthesis).

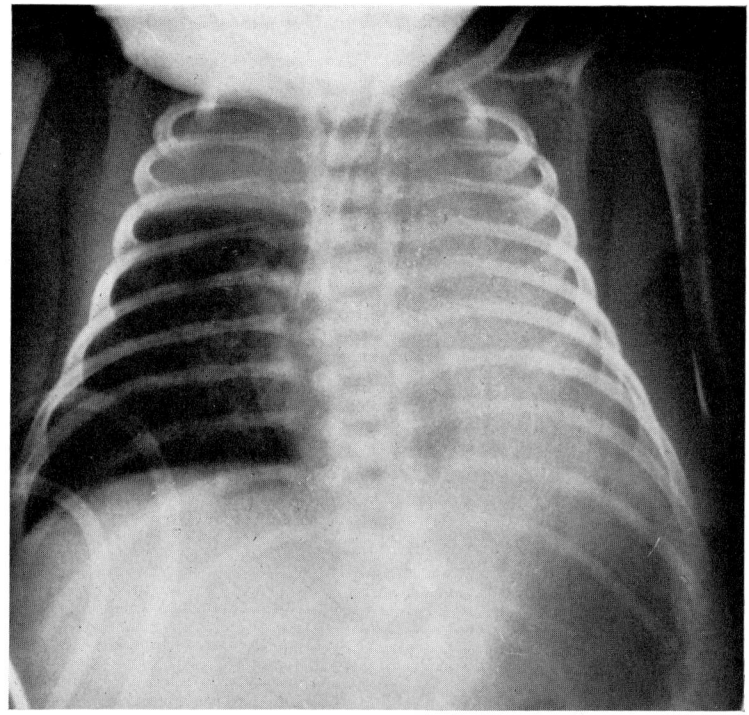

FIG. 10.5 An endotracheal tube has entered the right main bronchus, producing partial atelectasis of the right lung and complete collapse of the left. The right lower lobe shows compensatory emphysema.

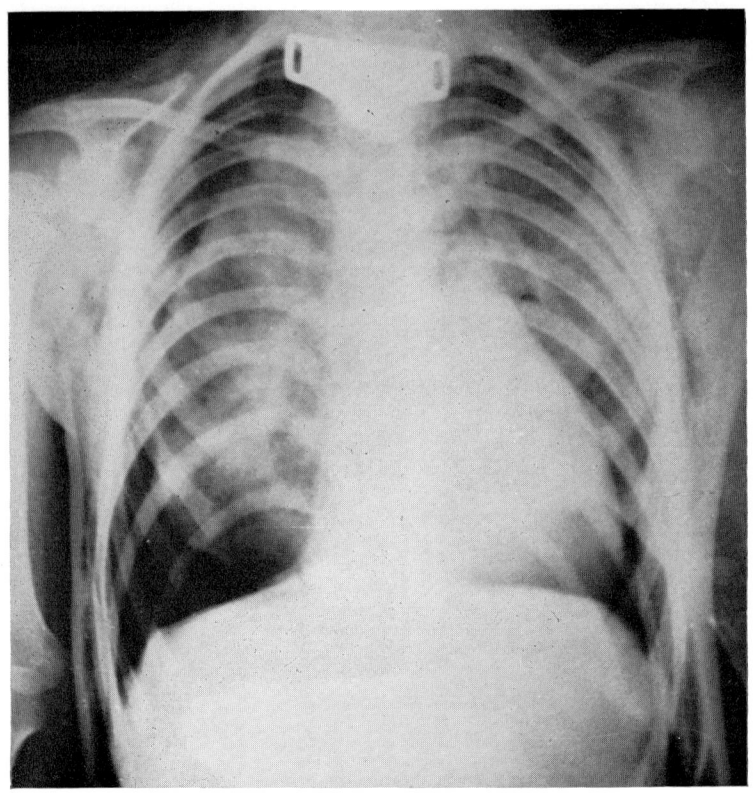
Fig. 10.6 Widespread leak of air into the tissues from a tracheostomy wound—an unusual complication. There is also air in the pleural cavities

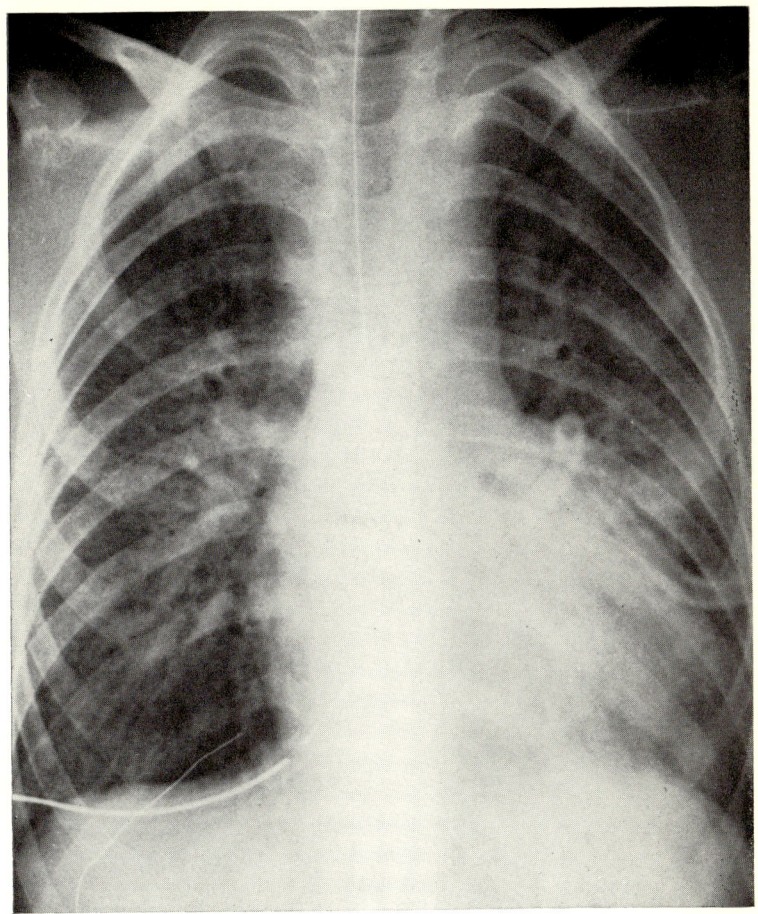

Fig. 10.7 A chest film taken after ventilation with over 80 per cent oxygen for five days, showing diffuse opacity in both lungs (reproduced by permission of the 'British Journal of Radiology').

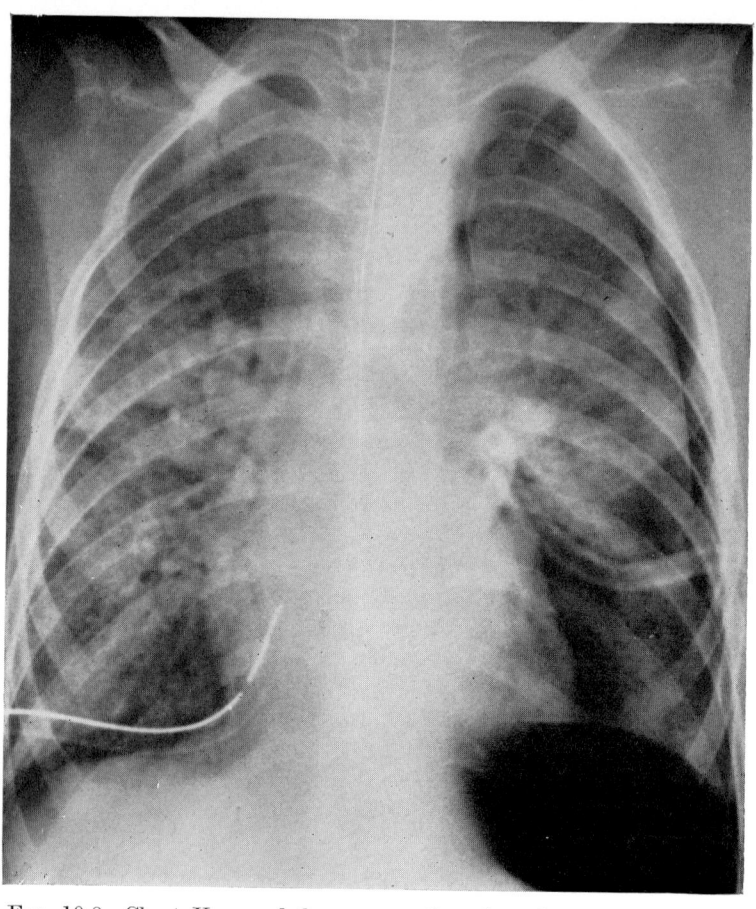

Fig. 10.8 Chest X-ray of the same patient four days later. The lung changes are more pronounced and alveolar rupture has caused a leak of air into the pleural cavities (reproduced by permission of the 'British Journal of Radiology').

CHAPTER
10

Radiological Investigations

The paediatric intensive therapy unit is specifically designed for the care of children with serious illnesses which require constant supervision and highly specialised treatment. Such care is most frequently needed for respiratory diseases, particularly bronchiolitis and laryngeal stridor and for neurological conditions that produce coma, such as status epilepticus and severe head injuries. Almost routinely, children who have undergone major thoracic surgery, especially for congenital heart lesions, are nursed in this type of unit for some time after operation. Many of these patients require artificial ventilation, usually with the aid of a plastic endotracheal tube. Occasionally tracheostomy is unavoidable if adequate ventilation is to be maintained.

Radiological examination is an integral part of the monitoring service which is an essential feature of intensive care, and that of the chest is particularly useful since so many of the patients have problems related to the respiratory tract.

RADIOGRAPHIC METHODS

Most patients in the I.T.U. are severely ill. Many receive artificial ventilation and have intravenous infusions and intercostal drainage tubes. It is therefore important that they should be disturbed as little as possible for radiographic examinations and it is clearly often impossible for them to travel to the X-ray department. Radiographic procedures are performed in the I.T.U. with various types of mobile

X-ray set (often referred to as 'portable' sets). These sets are not as powerful as modern departmental X-ray equipment which is energised by large generators and can produce a considerable quantity of radiation in a small fraction of a second. Some mobile units do have quite a high output but are of necessity large and bulky. It is often more convenient to use a smaller model, especially for paediatric examinations, and very satisfactory radiographs can be produced by a capable radiographer with this type of equipment. Besides technical skill, patience and gentleness are essential in handling very ill children who may have painful operation wounds.

The small mobile X-ray apparatus illustrated produces a current of about 25 milli-ampères through the X-ray tube, compared with a possible 1000 mA in a modern set in the X-ray department. The Kilovoltage which controls the penetrating qualities of the X-ray beam varies from 60 KV for chest radiographs in small children to 85 KV for children aged about 12 years. Exposure times are generally between 0·025 sec for a baby and 0·06 sec for a much larger child. A focus to film distance of 30 to 36 inches is used. All these factors are varied to suit the requirements of each individual case and depend on such conditions as whether the child is being ventilated or can hold his breath voluntarily, his level of consciousness and whether he is lying flat or able to sit up. Since all films in the I.T.U. are taken 'A.P.', that is to say, with the X-ray tube in front of the chest and the film cassette behind, and since focus to film distances are short, there is inevitably some magnification of the heart shadow in relation to the rest of the thorax, but this fact is taken into consideration when the films are interpreted. In the diagnostic X-ray department, older children are X-rayed with the tube behind them and the film in front, with a focus to film distance of 5 feet. This provides a much more accurate representation of the true size of the heart.

Chest radiographs are often taken in the I.T.U. with the patient lying flat. This is obviously necessary when an immediate post-thoracotomy film is required. The patient, who is often still sedated, is lifted with the least amount of disturbance and the cassette containing the film is slipped under the chest (Fig. 10.1).

This technique is also used for small infants who are critically ill and who are in incubators or receiving artificial ventilation. A nurse or attendant holds the child's extended arms alongside the head, keeping the chest straight (Fig. 10.2). This is an important point

Radiological Investigations

because even a small amount of rotation of the chest can give quite an erroneous impression (the mediastinum may appear displaced) and may invalidate the examination altogether.

When a baby is too ill to be moved from an incubator, the nurse can insert her hands through the port-holes to hold the child's arms alongside the head.

When children are fit enough to sit up, films are taken in this position with the cassette positioned correctly behind the chest (Fig. 10.3). The upright position has the advantage that the child may be able to inspire more deeply and the diaphragm can descend to a lower level, producing a more accurate picture of the heart and lungs.

The appearance of the heart and pulmonary vessels in children varies greatly according to the phase of respiration. Also, when films are taken in this way using a horizontal X-ray beam, fluid levels can be shown in the thorax when free air and fluid are present. A pneumoperitoneum can be shown as a dark line of air under the diaphragm when the child is sitting up. This may be important in diagnosing a perforated viscus or leaking anastamosis, though it must be remembered that some air can be seen in the abdomen for periods of 48 hours or more following laparotomy.

Radiological examination in the I.T.U. is greatly helped by the presence of easily accessible 13 amp sockets. It is important also to have a generous amount of space between beds, so that the X-ray set may be moved without disturbing patients and so that ventilators and monitoring equipment do not make it difficult to bring the X-ray set to the bed side.

Additional examinations in the I.T.U.

Examination of the abdomen is sometimes required when ileus or intestinal obstruction is suspected, and it is usually possible to produce satisfactory supine and erect films of the abdomen with the child's co-operation. It may be necessary to take radiographs to check the position of a tube in the duodenum or small intestine for the treatment of paralytic ileus or intestinal obstruction. When small infants with suspected intestinal obstruction are examined, it is a useful practice to take three radiographs—a supine, erect and a lateral film of the abdomen with the child inverted. The last film is especially useful in that it may show gas in the distal colon, helping to differentiate between intestinal obstruction and distension of the gut due to other causes.

Contrast Examinations

Only the most simple examinations using contrast media should be attempted in I.T.U. conditions, since this type of procedure is best performed under fluoroscopic control in the X-ray department. Occasionally, however, it is justifiable to perform a limited study with a small amount of contrast medium to determine, for instance, whether a jejunostomy or gastrostomy tube is correctly situated or to demonstrate the presence of a fistula. Limited examinations of this kind should be done only when specifically indicated and when subsequent treatment depends on the results of the examination. It should be remembered also that water-soluble contrast media attract fluid into the bowel and can produce a hypovolaemic state in small children. If there is any risk of aspiration, an inert contrast medium such as 'Lipiodol' should be used in preference to water-soluble media which can produce pulmonary oedema if aspirated into the lungs.

Radiological Aspects of Post-Operative Care

After thoracic operations, particularly cardiac surgery, a chest radiograph is essential as soon as the operation is completed to show that the lungs are well aerated and to exclude significant amounts of air or fluid in the pleural cavities. In the later post-operative period, chest radiographs are of value not only in assessing the state of the lungs and cardiovascular system but also to check the position of intercostal drainage tubes, naso-gastric catheters and endotracheal tubes when these are employed. Intercostal drainage tubes may be kinked or otherwise situated in a position that requires correction. Catheters for gastric aspiration or feeding frequently extend no further than the lower oesophagus and radiological examination is the most reliable method of determining their position with certainty. This is important when the stomach is distended with air after operation and gastric aspiration is required. It is essential after correction of oesophageal atresia to be sure that the feeding tube has

Radiological Investigations

been passed beyond the anastamosis into the stomach, otherwise injection of fluid down the tube may produce an anastamotic leak or aspiration into the lungs (Fig. 10.4).

The length of endotracheal tubes used in artificial ventilation must always be checked radiographically. In small children the lower end of the tube occasionally extends down as far as the carina and Fig. 10.5 shows an endotracheal tube which has entered the right main bronchus, causing partial collapse of the right lung and total collapse of the left. The tube must be repositioned without delay when this occurs.

After thoracic operations, fluid may collect in the mediastinum or the pleural cavities. Widening of the superior mediastinal shadow due to fluid is seen quite often after major cardiac operations and usually resolves after a few days. Post-operative pleural fluid also disappears quite rapidly as a rule; a persistent or increasing effusion may be a chylothorax, a rather uncommon complication due to injury to the thoracic duct or one of its main tributaries. It must be remembered that when chest radiographs are taken with the patient lying supine, pleural fluid may be concealed or may present an atypical appearance. There may be diffuse opacity of one half of the thorax due to a thin layer of fluid spread over the posterior chest wall. Fluid may also appear as a curved para-vertebral shadow which can be confusing, or it may form a peripheral layer around the lung. Conventional radiographs taken in an upright position show the upper edge of a pleural effusion as an oblique line extending upwards and outwards to the axilla.

Pulmonary atelectasis or consolidation is occasionally found after thoracotomy. When pulmonary lobes or segments become airless they shrink and often acquire characteristic shapes which assist in their recognition. The hilum of the lung may be higher or lower than normal, depending on the area affected. In major degrees of lung collapse the mediastinum is often displaced to the affected side and the diaphragm is elevated.

When lung is consolidated or contains fluid there is an area of opacity without reduction in volume. The bronchi in this area can remain patent and since they contain air they may be seen on the radiograph as an 'air bronchogram', the dark streaks of air being outlined against the dense background of solid lung. Not infrequently atelectasis of basal segments is found in children together with consolidation or fluid retention and this produces a combination of radiological features. Pulmonary oedema may be seen after cardiac operations and chest radiographs show diffuse hazy or 'miliary' density, often more pronounced in the central lung fields. Air in the chest wall is a common finding after thoracic operations and usually disappears quickly. An increasing amount of air in the chest wall, pleura or mediastinum, particularly after lung resection, demands attention.

Following surgery for cardiac lesions in infancy, the radiological appearance of the pulmonary vessels can provide useful information. After ligation of a ductus arteriosus, pulmonary vessels diminish in size due to reduction of blood flow through the lungs. Conversely, when the pulmonary circulation has been improved after operation for Fallot's tetralogy, increasing pulmonary vascularity is shown in the post-operative period.

After any major operation, dyspnoea can be caused by distension of the stomach by gas or swallowed air—a condition readily visible on chest radiographs. Gastric distension may occur during induction of anaesthesia. Post-operative pain and immobility can also be contributory factors.

Much of the information obtained from post-operative chest X-rays should be made available to the clinicians in charge of the I.T.U. without delay. Many clinicians prefer to view the films in the X-ray department soon after they have been processed. When this is not possible, it is often advisable for the radiologist to communicate information direct to the I.T.U., especially when the findings are unexpected or indicate a situation which needs prompt attention. In such cases, conveying information by means of typed reports alone is too slow a process, although this procedure should be observed in addition to the verbal report.

Radiological Aspects of Respiratory Diseases and Chest Injuries

The respiratory diseases which require intensive care fall into two main groups. First, there are those which cause obstruction of the air passages, such as laryngitis, tracheo-bronchitis, asthma and bronchiolitis. Second, there are conditions which cause respiratory failure by interfering with alveolar ventilation, such as extensive pneumonia, aspiration of toxic vapours and smoke, drowning, and pulmonary oedema due to a variety of causes. Upper respiratory tract infections may cause severe respiratory distress in small children, but as a rule chest radiographs show remarkably little of significance. However when there is partial laryngeal obstruction and stridor it is not uncommon to see evidence of tracheal collapse during inspiration, in the same way that a rubber tube can be made to collapse when suction is applied to one end with a syringe. Tracheal narrowing in inspiration must not be mistaken for organic stenosis; a film taken in expiration will show that the trachea returns to its normal width.

Asthma and bronchiolitis obstruct peripheral airways, mainly in expiration. The lungs become over-distended and appear more radiolucent than normal. The diaphragm is low and flattened; the antero-posterior diameter of the chest is increased and lateral chest films show an increased area of translucent lung in front of the heart shadow. There may be bulging of the intercostal spaces.

Thoracic injury can involve the chest wall or lung. Injury to the chest wall often causes a haemothorax which initially at least presents the appearance of a pleural effusion. Radiographs taken soon after rupture of a bronchus may show only a small pneumothorax but this can increase in size quite rapidly. A pneumothorax under tension can displace the mediastinum well over to the normal side in children and the pleural cavity on the affected side may become so distended that it bulges across the midline in a way not usually seen in adults.

Damage to the lung parenchyma can produce a variety of radiological appearances. There may be extensive mottled opacity due to pulmonary contusion. Occasionally a pulmonary haematoma is shown as a localised rounded opacity. The radiological appearances of trauma may be further complicated by pulmonary oedema which is reported to occur in some cases of hypovolaemic shock.

Radiological Aspects of Artificial Pulmonary Ventilation

The progress of patients treated by intermittent positive pressure ventilation is carefully observed. To prevent pulmonary complications the lungs are fully inflated at intervals, inspired gases are suitably humidified and the trachea is aspirated frequently to prevent accumulation of secretions. Ventilated patients should have chest radiographs at least once a day since in spite of all precautions, areas of atelectasis or fluid retention may develop in the lungs. The position of the endotracheal tube must be observed. When pulmonary disease produces stiffness of the lungs, known as reduced lung compliance, ventilation may become difficult and increased positive pressure may be required. When lung compliance is uneven, pressure required to ventilate the stiff areas may over-distend a more normal area of lung, leading to alveolar rupture and escape of air into the pleura or mediastinum. Normal lungs which are artificially ventilated (as in comatose states) may present the radiological appearance of over-distension since films are taken at the peak of inspiration. This should not be confused with pulmonary disease causing airways obstruction. When a tracheostomy has been performed, chest radiographs are of value in detecting evidence of lower respiratory infection which may develop in spite of careful management. There may of course be extensive tracheal and bronchial infection without an abnormal radiological appearance. Radiographs also provide a useful check on the position of the tracheostomy tube. An unusual complication of the operation of tracheostomy is leakage of air into the tissues around the wound and the air can spread freely into the neck and chest wall (see Fig. 10.6).

Artificial ventilation using high oxygen concentrations (80 per cent or more) for periods of several days has been shown to produce radiological and pathological changes which may develop within 60 to 70 hours after ventilation has begun. There is reduced lung compliance so that progressively higher positive pressures are required to maintain adequate ventilation. The radiological features of this condition are diffuse fine densities which are distributed fairly symmetrically in the lung fields. This at first resembles the appearance of some types of pulmonary oedema in which alveoli are filled with fluid, giving rise to numbers of very fine 'spots' on the chest radiograph.

As the disease progresses the radiographic opacity becomes more confluent and air-filled bronchi are seen against the dense background. An additional feature is the presence of round translucent areas representing dilated terminal air passages. Once established, this condition is usually fatal. At autopsy, the lungs are reddish in colour and of rubbery texture; histological examination shows thickening of alveolar walls and hyaline membranes in the alveoli

Radiological Investigations

and terminal bronchioles. Reports of this complication of artificial pulmonary ventilation suggest that the lowest possible oxygen concentrations should always be used (see Figs. 10.7 and 10.8).

The success of a diagnostic radiology service in the I.T.U. depends on a close liaison between radiologist and clinician. It is helpful if the radiologist is acquainted with the particular clinical problems of each case and he should be aware of the significance of apparently minor details such as the presence of a small pneumothorax after operation for oesophageal atresia which may be the first indication of an anastamotic leak. On the other hand, leaving air in the pleura after repair of a congenital diaphragmatic hernia is often necessary to maintain stability within the thorax because the lung on the side of the hernia is usually poorly developed and at first may not be able to expand enough to fill the available space. Exchange of such information is always in the best interests of the patient and makes a contribution towards efficient post-operative care.

As in other fields of diagnostic radiology it must be borne in mind that patients may be severely ill with respiratory diseases of which there is little radiological evidence. The clinical state of the patient must be taken into account and in interpreting films one must always bear in mind the conditions under which the examination was carried out. Observation of these principles will ensure that the best use is made of a diagnostic radiology service for the patients in an I.T.U.

CHAPTER 11

The Nurse in the I.T.U.

The nurse in the I.T.U. forms part of a specialised team consisting of nursing, medical and ancillary personnel who aim to provide the safest and most meticulous treatment and attention for the patients within their care. Because of the specialised management and supportive methods of treatment required to maintain life and aid recovery, the nurse requires knowledge and understanding of the use of modern monitoring equipment and certain special apparatus within her sphere. She should be of senior status—a state registered nurse of experience, able to reason objectively, to judge and be aware of rapidly changing situations. She must be capable of interpretation of data and of rapid decisive action. The state enrolled nurse can well play an important supportive role within the nursing team. Senior student nurses after two years experience should possibly spend time in a supplementary capacity working in the I.T.U. to gain training which would otherwise be lost to them. The degree of participation varies considerably and there is no universal norm. Overburdening student nurses with the responsibility of demanding and exacting tasks may do more harm than good, leading to apprehension, frustration and disenchantment, certainly not to better patient care. Shortage of nursing staff in an I.T.U. leads to added stress on the physical and emotional state required to withstand the strain of continually nursing critically ill patients.

The I.T.U. nurse is primarily responsible for continuous patient care and surveillance; she sees the overall picture, fulfils human needs, provides nursing care and comfort for her patients. She should be responsible for immediate patient care including the use and management of ventilators, monitors etc., but only following a period of learning and continuous experience within the unit. The continual changing pattern of patients within the unit highlights the need for a high ratio of permanent trained nursing staff to provide essential and desirable stability and continuity.

NURSING CARE

General nursing care in an I.T.U. differs little from that needed by any seriously ill medical or surgical patient. There may be added aids and devices to complement (complicate!) routine care but it must not be forgotten that careful continuous clinical observation by the nurse is essential.

One nurse per patient is required and indeed a second person is frequently needed so that routine procedures can be carried out effectively and smoothly causing least discomfort to the patient. Many patients are unable to communicate their needs for various reasons such as coma, drug-induced paralysis for controlled respiration, or patients who have a tracheostomy and therefore cannot speak. This should be borne in mind by the nurse in order to anticipate the patient's needs and alleviate discomfort.

Discussion pertaining to treatment should never be held before a child capable of understanding in part, with the possibility of causing apprehension. Appropriate verbal reassurance and competent but gentle handling will help allay fear. Nursing procedures required for these seriously ill patients must be balanced against the need for rest and quiet.

Unconscious patients are completely nurse dependent; although many aids and alarm systems are available the nurse should not rely entirely upon these but should use her eyes and ears to detect the unexpected happening. Observation of the level of consciousness, assessment of the adequacy of ventilation, and maintenance of a clear airway are paramount.

The health of the skin depends on maintenance of general cleanliness and the treatment of pressure areas. The skin should be kept dry, and this particularly applies to infants in high humidity incubators, who are more prone to infection and who are surrounded by an atmosphere favourable for bacterial growth.

Care of the mouth is an important procedure often made more difficult in small neonates by the presence of an endotracheal tube which contributes to increased salivation necessitating frequent treatment. In addition to aspiration of oral secretions, proper oral cleaning must be carried out routinely.

The eyes require special precautions in the unconscious state, or in patients who have been paralysed, in order to avoid ulceration of the cornea. The eyelids may be open and there is no blink reflex. Ulceration of the cornea is prevented by instillation of eye drops (methyl cellulose, normal saline, or chloramphenicol if the conjuctiva becomes infected), and the eyelids are kept closed by paraffin gauze secured over them with adhesive tape. Crusts and discharges are removed by swabbing with sterile normal saline.

In the ill patient it is essential to ascertain that urine is passed regularly and that the bladder does not become distended. Accurate recording of urine output is necessary, and this poses some difficulty in younger children and infants in whom it is usually necessary to collect urine in a plastic bag which is attached to the skin by an adhesive strip. The sensitive skin of infants may become sore with a risk of infection. If the unconscious patient is not automatically voiding urine an indwelling catheter may be necessary, with particular care to avoid the introduction of infection.

The care of the bowel is usually no problem in the short term I.T.U. patient. However, a prolonged period of recumbency, as in a ventilated patient, or of unconsciousness, may necessitate periodic evacuation of the bowel by enemata.

The patient's posture should be changed regularly every two hours (or perhaps more frequently if there are special indications) in order to prevent localised ischaemia of areas of the skin resulting in pressure sores. Generally speaking the unconscious patient should be nursed in the lateral position which is maintained by placing a pillow along the patient's back and flexing the upper leg to prevent pressure on the lower limb. The upper arm is placed slightly in front of the patient and the limbs are maintained in a natural position to avoid strain. Frequent turning from side to side is particularly important in cardiothoracic patients to assist drainage from the pleural cavities and to prevent the accumulation of secretions in any one part of the lungs. The physiotherapist plays an extremely important role in the care of patients in the I.T.U. in association with the nursing staff.

Collaboration between physiotherapist and nurse is important so that both are fully aware of the particular problems of each patient. The physiotherapist can show the nurse such procedures as 'shaking and vibration' and the application of pressure to the chest wall on expiration which assists in the expulsion of mucus, so that these manoeuvres can be carried out at a time when the physiotherapist may not be available. Passive movements of the limbs are important in order to avoid joint stiffening. This co-operation between physiotherapist and nurse ensures that a full régime of treatment can be obtained over the whole 24 hour period.

Nutrition and Fluid Balance

When gastro-intestinal feeding is tolerated it is preferable to provide adequate calories, vitamins and fluid intake by this route. This may be given via an intragastric tube inserted either through the nose or the mouth. Tube feeds may be intermittent or by slow continuous intragastric infusion so avoiding overdistension of the stomach and minimising the tendency to vomit or to embarrass respiration.

In the case of very small infants, feeding catheters are necessarily of fine gauge and therefore soft and flexible so that they may easily be dislodged. With all patients it is important to establish that the end of the tube is present in the stomach, but this is particularly important in the case of infants, as a feed given into the oesophagus may regurgitate and be inhaled. In addition to aspiration of the tube and testing the aspirate with litmus paper, it is important to use a feeding catheter with a radio-opaque sentinel line so that its position can be checked radiologically. If intermittent tube feeds are being employed the tube should be aspirated before each feed, and the nature of aspirate is described and its volume recorded. This is important in calculating the intake/output fluid balance.

If parenteral fluid replacement is required varying techniques are available. In the newborn a cannula may be inserted into the umbilical vein. It is preferable to spare veins in the neonate (as indeed in all children) by avoiding 'cut down' cannulation, and scalp vein infusion sets are available using very small needles with a flange so that the needle can be secured to the scalp by strapping. 'Cut down' cannulation of veins may be necessary if percutaneous cannulation is impossible. Subcutaneous infusion, assisted by the use of hyaluronidase, is a method rarely used with the severely ill patient in an I.T.U. Whatever technique is adopted it is essential to establish a continuous flow of fluid, and in the case of small infants it is usually necessary to ensure a slow flow rate in order not to overload the circulation. Low volume infusions may best be managed by the use of a constant slow infusion pump. With a slow infusion, clotting within the cannula is a risk and frequent observation of the rate of infusion is necessary. It may be advisable to restrict movement and protect the site of infusion chosen.

Intake/Output Recording

The collection of data relating to fluid balance and its recording is a task which frequently falls on to the junior nurse in the ordinary ward environment. It is essential in the I.T.U. that the nurse should appreciate that this vitally important information is necessary for the proper prescribing of fluid and electrolytes, and that unless measurements are accurate the patient's life may well be threatened.

All ways of taking fluid must be shown simultaneously on the same chart whether by mouth, nasogastric tube, gastrostomy, jejunostomy, intravenous infusion etc. It is essential to know the actual amount absorbed (this may vary from the amount meant to be given, for example, if a certain amount of a nasogastric tube feed is aspirated before the next feed is given). The type of intake must be displayed clearly. Intravenous fluids may vary from a dextrose solution to a mixture of dextrose with various electrolytes and the composition of the intravenous infusion must be stated clearly. Additions to the intravenous fluid (for example, potassium chloride added to the basic infusion solution) should be noted both on the chart and the intravenous infusion bottle. The nature of oral intake is important; for example, orange juice is a rich source of potassium, and this may be relevant to treatment. It is necessary to know the time of intake of fluid and when changes occur in the intake.

The output of fluid should take note of all routes of fluid loss. This will therefore involve urine, gastric aspirate and vomit, loss from intestinal fistulae, excessive sweating, and loss in faeces (for example, a child who has diarrhoea). It is obvious that some of these can only be approximate values and for this reason the most accurate control of fluid intake/output is by daily weighing either by conventional means or by frequent estimation of body weight on a weighing bed.

It is important that the intake/output chart should show 12 hour and 24 hour input and output totals and also that it should be easy to see the 'running balance', and whether there is a fluid excess or deficit.

Management of Chest Drainage

Following cardiothoracic surgery, drainage tubes may be inserted into the pericardial sac, the anterior mediastinum, and/or the pleural cavities. These are connected to underwater sealed drainage bottles as described in Chapter 12, a water seal being particularly necessary in the case of pleural drainage to prevent the passage of air into the pleural cavity and the production of a pneumothorax and collapse of the lung. The drainage bottle should initially contain a predetermined volume of fluid so that measurement of the increase of level will give an accurate recording of the volume of drainage. It is usually preferable to connect the drainage bottle to vacuum in order to promote satisfactory evacuation of fluid or air from the chest cavity.

The nurse must ensure that the chest tube is firmly fixed to the chest wall, and that no leakage is occurring between the tube and the stab wound in the skin. She must ensure that all connections remain air tight. The tube emerging from the chest should be 'milked', and also the connecting tubing to the drainage bottle, in order to prevent obstruction by clot. The drainage tube should be clamped periodically and the connecting tube disconnected in order to allow blood to drain from the connecting tube to the bottle. It is preferable to use two large artery forceps for this purpose, the jaws being protected by polythene tubing in order to avoid injuring the drainage tube itself. The tubing must be prevented from kinking or constriction and sufficient length of tube must be allowed for movement (changing the patient's position from side to side) but long loops of tubing below bed level must be avoided, which would allow blood to accumulate and clot. 'Milking' the tubes should be carried out frequently (for example, every 15 minutes soon after chest drainage has been instituted) and the volume of fluid lost through the drain each time this is done should be recorded. This gives accurate indication of the need for replacement of blood, for example. The nature of drainage should be recorded, whether blood, serum, pus etc., and the presence of any air leak should be noted. If vacuum assistance to drainage is *not* being employed the nurse should observe whether the fluid level in the tube in the drainage bottle fluctuates with respiration; absence of fluctuation may indicate that the drainage system has become blocked so that fluid or air may be accumulating within the chest.

Management of the Artificial Airway

Endotracheal intubation for mechanically assisted ventilation may be necessary for varying periods in severe illness and to aid recovery following major operations. Long term use of an artificial airway usually requires that tracheostomy should be performed. In either circumstance the loss of voice in the case of the conscious child, the presence of the tube, and the discomfort caused by aspiration of secretions is frightening. The child with an artificial airway is at risk and must never be left unsupervised. It is mandatory that the artificial airway must be kept clear of secretions, and crusting of secretions can be lethal. Artificial humidification may be achieved by instillation of normal saline drops into the tube, the use of high humidity air/oxygen tents, or by leading the inspired gas through special humidifiers.

Both an endotracheal tube and a tracheostomy tube must be fixed firmly in position. It is particularly important to avoid movement with naso-tracheal or oro-tracheal tubes as this has a risk of producing laryngeal oedema, while in the case of nasotracheal tubes undue movement against the nasal septum can produce severe ulceration. In the case of tracheostomy tubes these must be fixed with doubly-tied tapes secured by a knot which cannot readily be undone; individual practice will vary but the anchoring must be secure and safe. Active children will handle their tubes and may displace them unless they are firmly fixed. A soft collar under the tape will prevent chafing of the skin at the back of the neck.

If the artificial airway is connected to a ventilator, the ventilator tubing itself will be heavy and tend to pull the artificial airway out of place so that the ventilator tubing must be supported in an appropriate manner.

Varying types of tracheostomy tube are available; silver tubes are rarely used in I.T.U. practice, disposable plastic tubes being preferable. These are changed as often as necessary by the nursing staff. The area around the tracheostomy is cleaned as required and a sterile technique using disposable gloves is employed for tube changing. Tracheal dilators are neither necessary nor desirable at the bedside; with the type of tracheostomy performed in paediatric practice a dilator is not necessary for introduction of the tube, while attempts to use tracheal dilators in the small trachea of an infant will only lead to severe trauma.

Aspiration of an artificial airway requires two persons, one to restrain the child and the other to carry out the actual procedure. Forceps are not used for introduction of the catheter, but this is handled using sterile disposable gloves. Hand inflation of the lungs using a breathing bag connected to the endotracheal or tracheostomy tube and an oxygen line, together with instillation of normal saline drops, is carried out prior to suction. The aspirating catheter is used once only and then discarded. When passing the catheter down the artificial airway the vacuum line is compressed and is only released when suction is actually required. It is preferable to carry out 'withdrawal suction', and not to push the catheter up and down during the withdrawal phase which only causes mucosal trauma with a likelihood of infection and oedema. The technique should be carried out in a swift and gentle manner, and the whole procedure should take only the length of time that the nurse can hold her breath. She should remember that the suction catheter is blocking the patient's airway. Aspiration of the airway will frequently provoke coughing in infants and children and the older child will require reassurance as he may become frightened.

The presence of an artificial airway, particularly if this crosses the pharynx, may lead to some incoordination of swallowing and excessive oro-pharyngeal secretions. If these are allowed to accumulate some inhalation of secretions may occur. The oro-nasal area must therefore be aspirated as a clean procedure, without use of disposable gloves, and the aspirating catheter may be used more than once. *On no account must the trachea be aspirated using a catheter that has been introduced into the mouth.* Oral and pharyngeal suction must be carried out carefully to avoid irritation and injury. It is easy to inflict trauma during nasal suction, which should be carried out only when absolutely necessary.

Recordings of aspiration of the airway should show whether the aspirate is watery or thick, the amount obtained (little or copious), the colour whether clear, purulent or blood stained, the frequency of treatment, whether physiotherapy has been carried out, and whether saline drops have been instilled into the airway or special chemotherapeutic measures have been adopted.

Management of Monitoring Cannulae

A plastic cannula may be inserted into a large vein for recording central venous pressure. Common sites are the superior vena cava via the internal jugular vein, or the inferior vena cava via the internal saphenous vein or femoral vein. It is the nurse's responsibility to ensure that the cannula remains patent and does not kink, to note any fluid administered by this route, and to record the level of venous pressure at regular intervals. If the central venous pressure is being measured on an oscilloscope via a transducer, the mean pressure should be recorded. If, however, the pressure is being measured by means of a saline manometer the nurse should note that some oscillation takes place with respiration and the mid-point of the swing should be taken as the level.

Arterial cannulation is employed in order to record continuously systolic and diastolic pressure, and usually the radial, brachial or femoral artery is selected. The nurse must see that the cannula is secure, as an inadvertently displaced cannula will lead to arterial bleeding. The cannula must be kept patent by syringing with a small quantity of heparinised saline at regular intervals. The arterial cannula is also used to obtain arterial blood samples for acid/base determinations and blood gas studies, and the first aspiration should be discarded as it will be contaminated with the heparinised saline used for irrigation. Flow of blood from the artery along the cannula will eventually lead to deposition of clot along its walls and interfere with accurate pressure recording, and a 'damped' or unexpectedly low blood pressure recording should be an indication to syringe the cannula in order to ensure its patency. The arterial blood pressure recordings are noted on the appropriate chart as often as deemed necessary.

Observations and Data Presentation

At the commencement of intensive care of an individual patient

Respiration

If spontaneous respiration is present the rate, depth and regularity of breathing should be noted and particular attention paid to the early recognition of respiratory difficulty. If controlled ventilation using mechanical assistance is necessary, a chart should be kept showing the rate of ventilation, inspiratory/expiratory ratio, pressure attained on the manometer on the ventilator, flow rate of the inspiratory gases, P_{O_2}, P_{CO_2}, and the patient's colour. An apnoea alarm is a useful aid to monitoring respiration in premature infants.

Pulse

The nurse must ensure that *all* peripheral pulses are readily palpable. She should note the volume and regularity of the pulse and should record any discrepancy between the heart rate and the peripheral pulse rate. A useful aid to changes in pulse rate is the use of a cardioscope with an audible 'bleep'; changes in rate and rhythm can then be detected both visually and audibly.

Arterial blood pressure

Continuous recordings of arterial pressure by arterial cannulation and display on an oscilloscope should be complemented by recording of systolic pressure by palpation and the use of a sphygmomanometer, the cuff of which is left in position in order to avoid repeated disturbance of the patient. This is important to give a base line of arterial pressure for when arterial cannulation is discontinued, and it is important to note that direct and sphygmomanometer pressures are often not identical. Arterial pressure recording gives important information with regard to adequate cardiac output.

Central venous pressure

This is important in considering the state of the circulating blood volume and also in assessing cardiac function. The central venous pressure will be low when there is hypovolaemia, and high if there is right ventricular failure or compression of the heart by fluid or blood clot.

Temperature

It is important that body temperature should be controlled within normal limits, and recording of temperature may be continuous, via an oesophageal or rectal thermocouple attached to an electrothermometer, or intermittent, using a clinical thermometer. It is important to state the site of recording of temperature. Skin temperatures are unreliable and it is preferable to measure the 'core' temperature. Continuous monitoring of temperature is particularly important in the case of patients who require cooling because of hyperpyrexia, and also in those who require warming because they are hypothermic. In the case of premature infants, nursing is preferably carried out in a servo-controlled incubator in which the baby's temperature and the incubator temperature are mutually adjusted; most of these incubators rely on recording the infant's temperature by means of a skin electrode (which does not necessarily reflect 'core' temperature), or by means of a rectal thermocouple, which may give inaccurate readings because of insulation by faeces, so that it is preferable also to measure the infant's temperature periodically by more conventional means.

Data presentation

Records of temperature, pulse, arterial pressure, central venous pressure and respiration are usually made in graph form on a chart thus making any change readily seen. Each type of recording should have its own colour marking which makes variations of pattern more distinguishable. It is the responsibility of the nurse to make sure that recordings are accurate, neat and clearly marked at the appropriate time so that they are easily understood not only by her but by others. The individual patient's records are preferably kept on a lectern-type stand at the bedside which makes for easy writing and display.

Collection of specimens

It is frequently the nurse's task to obtain specimens for ward and laboratory examination. Thus urine may be kept for ordinary ward testing including the measurement of specific gravity, and may also be required for biochemical examination of the 24 hours output of electrolytes and urea.

Any specimen required for laboratory examination *must* be dispatched in the appropriate receptacle which may contain a special preservative.

Blood specimens are required both for haematological investigation and biochemical examination including Astrup determination of acid/base balance and measurement of Po_2.

In many instances information required by examination of material from a patient in an I.T.U. is needed urgently, as the results will often modify treatment over the next few hours. There must therefore be no delay in sending specimens to the appropriate department. The specimen must be clearly labelled with the patient's name in full, the date and time at which the material was obtained, the hospital registration number, the nature of the specimen and the fact that it has come from the I.T.U. It must be accompanied by a request form legibly completed and indicating the appropriate investigations required. If necessary the laboratory is warned that the specimen is being dispatched.

Early communication of laboratory findings is vital. It is important that correct information is recorded, and verbal messages by telephone must be repeated back to the person giving the information and written clearly before being transmitted to medical staff. While verbal messages are useful to avoid the delay in receiving typed reports through the usual channels, the latter should also be obtained as a check on the verbal communication.

If it is anticipated that certain laboratory investigations may be likely outside normal working hours, it is helpful to inform laboratory staff accordingly as this promotes a successful and co-operative working relationship.

THE NURSE IN THE EMERGENCY SITUATION

The I.T.U. nurse must be watchful and vigilant in patient care, as changes in the patient's condition can be sudden and deterioration rapid, leading to collapse. She must have adequate training in the procedure to be adopted in the event of cardio-respiratory arrest. It is imperative that she should remain calm, think clearly, act quickly, and summon medical help, using the emergency call system.

External haemorrhage is rarely seen but, if occurring, should be managed by direct pressure if possible. Most acute emergencies are associated with respiratory obstruction or arrest, or falling cardiac output or cardiac arrest.

The nurse must first ascertain whether pulse and/or respiration are absent. The patient must be put flat and the upper airway examined and cleared if necessary by suction. The jaw must be held forward and, if breathing has ceased, oxygen administered using a face mask and breathing bag attached to an oxygen line, a Guedel airway being inserted into the mouth if necessary. Distension of the stomach must be avoided and this may require the passage of a large stomach tube. Inadequate cardiac output (even if the E.C.G. still shows a reasonably regular tracing) is treated by external cardiac massage as described in Chapter 18. The resuscitation trolley must be brought to the bedside for the use of the duty anaesthetist. When relieved by the medical staff the nurse should ensure that relevant drugs are available for administration and also that an intravenous infusion can be set up or that an existing infusion is preserved if possible. Infants will have to be taken out of their incubators, and it is important to avoid too much heat loss while resuscitation is being carried out, either by use of an infra-red lamp or thermostatically controlled warming blanket.

The Patient's Relatives

The nurse in the I.T.U. is called upon to maintain a close understanding with the relatives of the children in her care. Although a child may be unconscious, and the small infant does not recognise his parents, many adults feel the need to remain with their children and this must be accepted and provided for, although it must be stressed that prolonged visiting, as occurs in a general paediatric ward, will not be possible as it interferes with the amount of nursing and medical care required. Parental anxiety and fear for the child's well-being is great and explanation of special equipment used, the child's progress, and changes in management are all necessary. If the child is making satisfactory progress towards recovery appropriate reassurance must be given to his parents, but it is equally important to give adequate warning of deterioration. Parents may experience psychological difficulties over a prolonged period of severe illness between their commitment to family and home on the one hand, and attendance on the ill child on the other. The nurse must try to appreciate these problems and allow for visiting at any mutually convenient time.

The death of any child is a great loss to the family, and the psychological stress following a severe illness managed in the I.T.U., the child being surrounded by monitoring equipment and possibly being paralysed and attached to a ventilator, may be much greater than when death occurs at home or in the ordinary ward. The nurse, realising her limitations, should do everything possible to provide comfort and reassurance by her care and consideration for the child during his illness.

Intensive care is a demanding, yet stimulating, sphere of nursing, but it must not be forgotten that it is in the individual patient's comfort and care that the nurse gains her reward.

CHAPTER

12

Care of Respiratory Problems

DIAGNOSIS OF RESPIRATORY DISEASE

Symptoms and Signs

Respiratory disease necessitating hospital admission either has an acute onset, or is an acute exacerbation of a chronic disease. The rapidity of onset, rate of progress, possible inhalation of a foreign body, or a sudden coughing fit while eating, are all important, as is the presence of cough, whether or not it is productive, the presence of cyanosis, or noisy breathing. In the infant, nasal obstruction may cause difficulty with feeding.

Observation of the patient must include pulse and respiratory rate, temperature, posture, and note of obvious respiratory difficulty, giving intercostal recession, use of accessory muscles of inspiration, and working of alae nasi. The shape of the chest, and presence of clubbing will provide evidence of long-standing disease. Restlessness and air hunger may be observed, and often babies with respiratory distress will lie with the back and neck extended (opisthotonus) but without neck rigidity. The colour of the lips and mucous membranes should be observed, with the child both in and out of oxygen if cyanosed. Peripheral oedema may indicate associated cardiac failure.

If the patient has noisy breathing, stridor and wheezing should be carefully distinguished. *Wheezing* occurs in asthma, or bronchiolitis, is due to bronchospasm, and is most marked on expiration. It may be associated with overdistended lungs and the use of accessory muscles

Care of Respiratory Problems

of respiration. Auscultation reveals rhonchi, mainly expiratory, of varying pitch, according to the degree of bronchial narrowing. The disappearance of the rhonchi, with a silent chest indicates worsening of the spasm. *Stridor* is usually inspiratory, and is due to pharyngeal or laryngeal obstruction. If severe, it is associated with indrawing of the tissues of the neck, and of the sternum, on inspiration. There is often poor air entry into the lungs, and expiration is not difficult. The associated cough is barking and non-productive. A very ill child with a sudden onset of a rather low-pitched stridor may be suffering from epiglottitis, and rapid diagnosis is imperative, as death may occur suddenly. Gentle depression of the tongue reveals a large red epiglottis, but this examination should be carried out only where intubation equipment is at hand, because sudden respiratory obstruction may occur. These children have a septicaemia, and should be treated with antibiotics, after blood has been taken for culture.

Investigations

X-ray of the chest may reveal disease of the lungs and pleura, and will also to a certain extent show patency of the airway, especially if a lateral view of the neck is taken.

X-ray screening of the pharynx and larynx is useful in the differential diagnosis of stridor, and screening of the chest will demonstrate obstructive emphysema, if unilateral.

Blood gas studies are invaluable in the diagnosis of respiratory failure and in following the progress of treatment. Arterial blood is preferable, measuring $P\text{co}_2$ and $P\text{o}_2$. If this is unobtainable, the Astrup measurement may be made on capillary blood, drawn from a warm, vasodilated, heel or finger. It is useless and misleading to attempt this estimation on blood drawn, after great pressure, from a vasoconstricted area, when peripheral circulatory failure is present. The normal range for $P\text{co}_2$ is 36 to 44 mm Hg and for $P\text{o}_2$ is 95 to 100 mm Hg (breathing air).

Haemoglobin and packed cell volume measurements will show polycythaemia in the chronically hypoxic patient.

Bacterial examination and culture of the sputum, or a throat swab, should be routine, and a blood culture may be helpful.

Measurement of tidal and minute volumes, FVC, FEV_1 etc. may be of use in older children.

Laryngoscopy and bronchoscopy are useful both for diagnosis and treatment.

Respiratory Failure

This condition is said to be present if the $P_a\text{co}_2$ is above the normal limit, or if the patient is hypoxic, due to respiratory disease. Arbitrary levels at which treatment should be begun cannot be given, because blood gas studies should always be used in conjunction with the general condition of the patient, and the natural history of the disease.

Causes of respiratory failure

1. Depression of respiratory centres
   e.g. head injury,
   prolonged hypoxia,
   opiate overdose,
   barbiturate overdose.
2. Impaired function of motor nerves, or neuromuscular junctions
   e.g. poliomyelitis,   ⎫ bulbar palsy
   peripheral neuritis,   ⎬ often associated
   Guillain-Barré   ⎪ with respiratory
   syndrome,   ⎭ failure
   myasthenia gravis.
3. Disease of respiratory muscles
4. Limitations of movement of thoracic cage
   e.g. fractured ribs,
   flail chest,
   sclerodema,
   sclerema,
   elevation of diaphragm
   e.g. due to abdominal
   distension,
   status epilepticus.
5. Compression of the lung
   e.g. pleural effusion,
   pneumothorax.

6. Airway obstruction (i) upper
   e.g. epiglottitis (H. influenzae),
   laryngotracheobronchitis (virus),
   traumatic laryngeal oedema,
   foreign body,
   'congenital laryngeal stridor',
   congenital laryngeal web etc.,
   Pierre-Robin syndrome.
   Airway obstruction (ii) lower
   e.g. bronchiolitis (virus),
   asthma,
   acid aspiration syndrome of Mendelson,
   obstructive emphysema.
7. Pulmonary disease (i) decrease in functioning lung tissue
   e.g. pneumonia,
   atelectasis,
   fibrocystic disease.
   Pulmonary disease (ii) decreased compliance
   e.g. restrictive disease,
   pulmonary vascular
   congestion.
   Pulmonary disease (iii) emphysema

TREATMENT OF RESPIRATORY DISEASE

The inhalation of a foreign body must be excluded, and the degree of respiratory failure estimated from pulse and respiratory rate, general appearance and condition, and $P_a\text{CO}_2$ measurement. This assessment must be repeated to determine efficacy of treatment.

Increased viscosity of bronchial secretions should be prevented by keeping the patient well hydrated, by intravenous therapy if necessary, and by provision of a moist atmosphere. Drugs to cause bronchodilatation, such as isoprenaline, orciprenaline, hydrocortisone, and to loosen bronchial secretions, such as acetyl cysteine, may be given as aerosols if desired. Muscle relaxants may also be given by this route.

A moist atmosphere is provided normally by nebulisation of water, either into an incubator, into a plastic tent, or by a machine which directs a stream of nebulised water at the patient, e.g. the 'Croup-aire'.* Oxygen or air can be used as the vehicle. Tents tend to get hot, and ice may be needed to cool the water. Adequate elimination of carbon dioxide from the tent is essential.

Oxygen should be given as necessary, but only enough to improve arterial oxygen saturation, as a high oxygen intake may damage the lungs, and the eyes in premature babies. Care must be taken with administration of oxygen in chronic respiratory disease, as carbon dioxide narcosis may supervene.

Cautious sedation may be very helpful, but a careful watch must be kept on the pulse and respiratory rate, as restlessness may be a sign of hypoxia and impending respiratory failure.

Drugs such as antibiotics and antispasmodics, and those for the treatment of cardiac failure, are used where indicated.

Physiotherapy is often helpful, especially as it encourages coughing, and therefore, clearing of bronchial secretions. Pharyngeal suction may stimulate coughing in young children but it should always be remembered that the suction is pharyngeal, not endotracheal.

Positioning of the head sometimes helps to lessen respiratory obstruction in such conditions as the Pierre-Robin syndrome and 'congenital laryngeal stridor'. In both, the larynx is normal, and the obstruction due to a relatively large tongue and small jaw in the former, and to muscular incoordination in the latter. If the jaw and tongue can be held forward, the obstruction is often lessened, and a tracheostomy may be avoided. A special frame is available, on which the baby is nursed prone, with the jaw hanging. The baby has to be heavily sedated to tolerate this position, and fed by nasogastric tube. Congenital stridor may be lessened by passing a strap under the chin and suspending the baby from the head of the incubator, by a slight head-up tilt. Heavy sedation is again needed, but this method has been used successfully.

If sputum retention occurs, and causes respiratory embarrassment, *endotracheal suction* after intubation is a useful procedure. If the sputum is very thick and sticky, bronchial lavage with normal saline is employed, always remembering that fluid is absorbed very rapidly from the bronchial tree, and overloading of the circulation is possible in babies. Amounts up to 10 ml can be used, depending on the size of the patient. This can be very beneficial in asthma. If instituted early

* Manufactured by Airshields (U.K.) Ltd., Shoeburyness, Essex.

Care of Respiratory Problems

enough, it will assist the dilution of gastric acid which is so harmful to the bronchial tree after inhalation of vomit.

Respiratory stimulants, such as nikethamide, should *never* be used. They are non-specific cerebral stimulants, which increase oxygen need, and their effects are exerted for a much shorter time than the disease process, so giving no lasting advantage. They may cause convulsions, especially in the hypoxic patient.

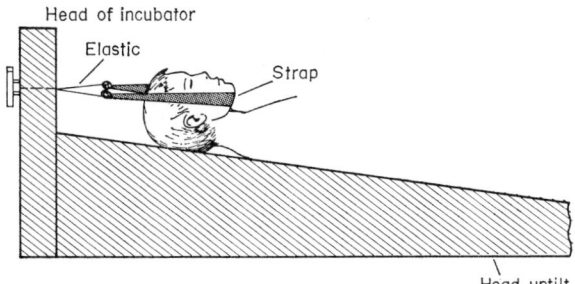

FIG. 12.1 Head harness for congenital laryngeal stridor.

If improvement is not obtained by the methods outlined above, and if respiratory failure is present, *intubation of the trachea* should be carried out. If the situation is urgent, or the general condition of the patient is poor, this may be done without sedation, but if there is time, sedation or general anaesthesia is preferable, in order to avoid trauma. In an emergency it is better to insert the tube by the oral route, as it is quicker and less traumatic. However, for long-term use, an oro-tracheal tube tends to be unstable, and is easily bitten, so that later, under general anaesthesia, a naso-tracheal tube should be substituted, or a tracheostomy carried out, depending on the circumstances. An emergency tracheostomy without anaesthesia is unnecessary, and indeed dangerous, except in the rare instance when intubation is impossible.

Such provision of an *artificial airway* may be sufficient to improve the condition of the patient, e.g. in upper airway obstruction, asthma, or crushed chest. Its advantages are that any upper airway obstruction is bypassed; the anatomical dead space is reduced (more so by tracheostomy), so alveolar ventilation is increased; it facilitates tracheal suction, and the application of moisture, oxygen and antispasmodics. Its disadvantages are that the efficiency of coughing is reduced, the patient cannot speak, and the danger of introduction of infection is great. By far the greatest disadvantage is that the natural humidification of inspired gases provided by the nose is bypassed, and unless a properly humidified atmosphere is provided, bronchial secretions become thick and inspissated, and the cilia of the cells of the bronchial mucosa stop working, so sputum retention occurs.

The decision whether to use *endotracheal intubation or tracheostomy* is influenced by many factors. Certainly a red rubber tube must not be left *in situ* for more than twelve hours, as it is irritant to the tissues, but plastic tubes may be left much longer. The actual safe time is controversial, but as a general rule should be no longer than five days in an older child, and ten days in an infant. If it can be predicted that an artificial airway will be needed for longer than this, then tracheostomy should be done early.

Prolonged endotracheal intubation

As has been stated, the nasal route is to be preferred in children, for greater stability and less liability to kinking. The *size of tube* must be very carefully selected. The size of the tube which should just fit through the larynx should be estimated from the formula

$$\text{size in mm} = \frac{\text{age}}{4} + 4 \cdot 5$$

and then a tube selected either a half size or preferably a whole size smaller. There will be a leak back around such a tube if pressure is put on the lungs, but this does not matter in practice, and can be compensated for if ventilation is required. Inflatable cuffs are not used on small tubes, because this increases the external diameter of the tube, and only allows one of much smaller lumen to be used, thereby increasing resistance to gas flow. However, a cuff may be preferred in older children, and is usual in adults, but these tubes are usually inserted orally.

Too large a tube will hold the vocal cords widely apart and will also encourage subglottic oedema, both of which factors predispose to the occurrence later of subglottic stenosis, a complication which is very difficult to treat. Trauma also predisposes to this complication, and therefore tubes should be kept as still as possible, and changed only when necessary. The tube is fixed to the face with adhesive tape, or

Care of Respiratory Problems

held in place by a head harness, the exact method being immaterial, provided the tube is held still, and damage to the nose and face avoided. The length of the tube should be carefully judged so that it is well into the trachea, but does not sit at the carina or down one bronchus. This can be checked by X-ray.

Other *complications* of prolonged intubation are ulceration of the nasal septum, difficulty in breathing through very narrow tubes (2·5 mm and 3·0 mm) and difficulty of adequate suction down such tubes because of small calibre and length. Laryngeal oedema may occur on extubation, and may require re-intubation for its relief. A short course of steroid therapy is thought to help prevent this rebound oedema.

The use of prolonged intubation avoids the neck scar left after tracheostomy, and can be very useful for bypassing upper airway obstructions, and for ventilation of the lungs. There are three types of tube which may be used:

1. A *plain plastic tube with a nasal/oral bevel*. An endotracheal connector should be left in the end to facilitate inflation of the lungs after suction.
2. A *Jackson-Rees* plastic tube*, which has a cross-piece, open in all four directions, for the connection of a ventilator. Suction is carried out down the central limb.

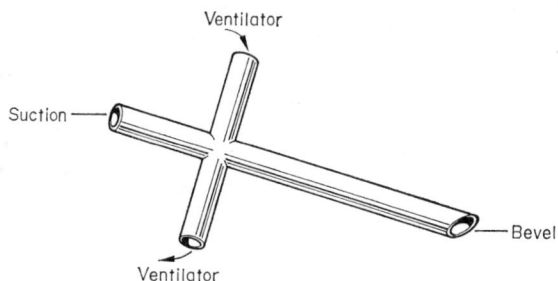

FIG. 12.2 Jackson-Rees tube.

This tube can be useful for artificial ventilation, but it has the disadvantages of a relatively thick wall, and the fact that it must be cut to the right length at the tracheal end, so that it may be difficult to avoid a sharp edge.

* Manufactured by Portex Ltd., Hythe, Kent.

3. *Warne 'Riplex'* neonatal tube*, which has a relatively large diameter down to the last inch, this having the correct diameter for the larynx. There are four sizes, from 12 to 18 F.G. These tubes are used orally, and are unlikely to kink, but are easily displaced. It is unwise to avoid displacement by pushing the tube firmly into the larynx, as the wider part may press on the vocal cords and subglottic area.

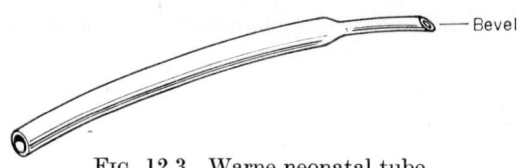

Fig. 12.3 Warne neonatal tube.

Tracheostomy

If an artificial airway is going to be required for a long time, then a tracheostomy should be done early. It should be performed in the operating theatre under general endotracheal anaesthesia. Operating on a struggling hypoxic child leads to excessive bleeding from distended neck veins and may cause surgical emphysema, either from damage to the pleura, or from sucking air into cut tissues with the strong inspiratory effort. The neck should be extended over a sandbag and the head held straight. A small transverse incision is normally made in the skin, and the thyroid isthmus divided. The incision in the trachea must be made below the first tracheal ring, otherwise laryngeal stenosis occurs. On the other hand, if the incision is too low, it will disappear behind the sternum when the neck is flexed, causing displacement of the tube. It is seldom necessary to suture the skin wound. The type of tracheal incision may be one of four (Fig. 12.4).

Each type has been used successfully, but all have some disadvantage. In the first forty-eight hours, until the track is well-formed, tracheostomy tubes can be difficult to replace, except in the flap type, where tube changing is easy initially and displacement of the tube into the tissues of the neck is unlikely. This makes this type of tracheostomy very safe. Its main disadvantages are that it may cause forward displacement and kinking of the trachea, and a granuloma may form around the stitch connecting the flap to the skin, but on the whole it is very satisfactory for all ages.

* Manufactured by William Warne and Co. Ltd., Barking, Essex.

Care of Respiratory Problems

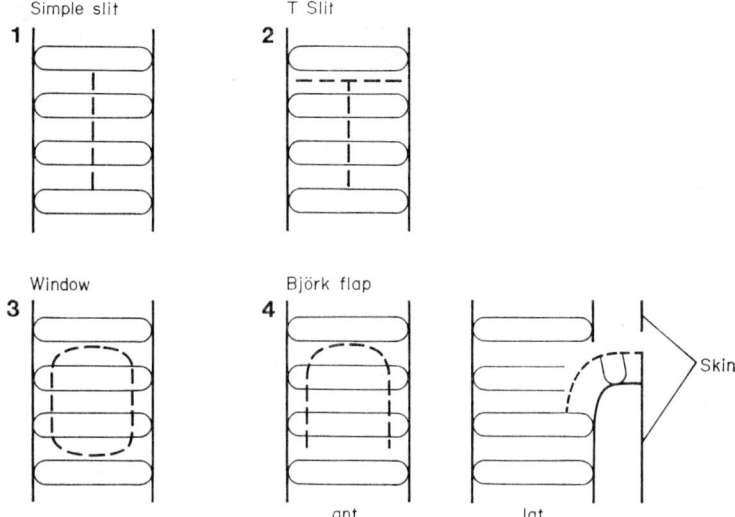

FIG. 12.4 Types of tracheal incision.

With the slit types of tracheostomy, some tracheal distortion is inevitable to form a round opening for the tube, worse in a narrow trachea. A displaced tube can be extremely difficult to replace soon after operation, especially in infants, where tracheal dilators cannot be used as they fill the tracheal lumen, and may split it. It is easy to insert the tube into the tissues of the neck and cause surgical emphysema.

This latter difficulty also occurs with the window type, and a defect is left in the trachea after decannulation, to which the skin will become attached, leaving an ugly scar.

There are three basic types of tracheostomy tube:

1. *red rubber*—these are irritant to tissues and should no longer be used.
2. *silver*—these have inner and outer cannulae for ease of cleaning, but the lumen is too small in infants, and the inner tube not used. They are only rarely used.
3. *plastic*—(i) with inflatable cuff. These are not made in small sizes, as the cuff decreases the possible lumen size, but are better in older children, to provide a seal.

(ii) plain tubes without cuff.

(a) tubes of 'Portex'* type which have a very narrow orifice, and insertion of a connector for inflation of the lungs narrows this still more, causing resistance to gas flow.

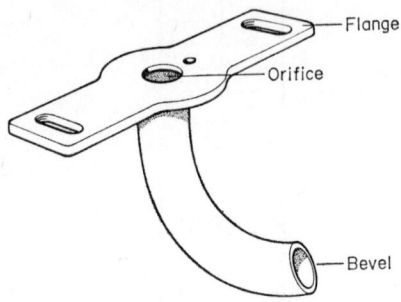

FIG. 12.5 'Portex' tracheostomy tube.

(b) Great Ormond Street infants' pattern.† These tubes are designed to take the same size of connector for all tube sizes, and the orifice at the flange is larger than the rest of the tube, so these are preferable for breathing spontaneously.

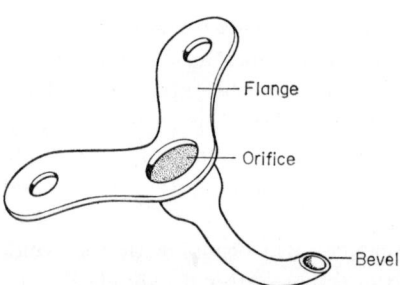

FIG. 12.6 Great Ormond Street tube.

A foolproof method of securing tracheostomy tubes is essential. It must be remembered that the tapes should be tied with the neck flexed, as in this position the neck is narrowest, otherwise the tube may slip out when the head is brought forwards. The tapes must be tied tightly and a soft collar under them is more comfortable. These tapes must not be tied in a bow, but must be knotted in such a fashion that scissors are needed to remove the tube.

* Manufactured by Portex Ltd., Hythe, Kent.
† Manufactured by J. G. Franklin & Son Ltd., London.

Care of Respiratory Problems

Tracheostomy shares with endotracheal intubation the disadvantages of lack of natural humidification, inability to cough properly or to speak, increased susceptibility to infection, and possible death from asphyxia, if the tube becomes blocked or displaced, but it also has its own problems.

Surgical emphysema may occur, especially if the tube becomes blocked. Obstruction of the orifice can happen easily in babies, who have short necks and double chins, and careful positioning of the head and shoulders, together with continuous supervision, is needed. As children get older they become more capable of protecting their own airway. Stricture of the trachea is a complication, which usually occurs at the site of an inflated cuff. It is a difficult condition to treat, but strictures have been successfully dilated or resected.

The larynx may become incompetent after tracheostomy, and saliva and food may be inhaled. Some babies seem to lose coordination of the larynx and become incapable of breathing if the tracheostomy is closed. For this reason, decannulation can be a prolonged procedure. Use of the larynx should be encouraged by fenestration of the tube, use of the speaking valve, and gradual blocking of the opening.

Management of an artificial airway

1. As has already been mentioned, *firm fixation* of the tube is mandatory, and excessive movement must be avoided—i.e., ventilator tubes must be fully supported and not allowed to drag.

2. Tracheostomy tubes should be changed routinely every one or two days, but endotracheal tubes may only be changed if they slip out or become obstructed, because routine changing must involve some trauma, with resultant laryngeal damage. Obstruction of an artificial airway can be fatal, unless immediately recognised.

The obstructed tube should always be removed. Another should be substituted as soon as possible. There must always be a spare tracheostomy tube beside the bed. In the case of an endotracheal tube, inflation of the lungs should be carried out by face mask until the tube can be replaced.

3. *Inspired gases* must be fully *humidified* to prevent crusting of secretions. If this does occur, it may be helped by the installation of water or normal saline down the tube. Sodium bicarbonate solution is irritant to the trachea and should not be used.

4. *Aspiration of the tube* should be performed every hour, or as often as is necessary—e.g. when secretions can be heard bubbling in the tube. The only exception to this rule is when frank pulmonary oedema is present. In this case some believe it is better not to suck on the lungs, because this may increase the oedema.

Aspiration *must* be performed with a strictly aseptic technique, by using either disposable plastic sterile gloves, or a pair of sterile forceps, to direct the suction catheter. If the catheter touches anything outside the tube it is unsterile, and asepsis cannot be maintained by a person working alone with a struggling child. It is always advisable to have two people for each aspiration if this is possible. A suction catheter must be selected, of such a size as to pass readily down the tube, leaving ample space for air to flow beside it but it must aspirate the bronchial tree effectively. With the narrow tubes necessarily used in babies, there is some danger of causing pulmonary collapse because of the need to use relatively large suction catheters, thereby exerting suction directly on the lungs. For this reason, hand inflation of the lungs is practised routinely after suction. Suction is withheld during introduction of the catheter either by kinking it, or leaving a Y connector in the circuit with one limb open. When suction is required, the open limb is occluded. Suction should not be left on for longer than fifteen seconds, because of the danger of producing hypoxia.

5. *To detect* introduction of any *infection* into the trachea, suction catheters are cultured routinely, usually once weekly, or more often if needed.

If respiratory failure persists, in spite of the introduction of an artificial airway, and perhaps bronchial lavage, then *artificial ventilation of the lungs* will be required. It must be emphasized that this seldom treats the original condition, but only allows time for that condition to improve. The exception is pulmonary oedema, which is decreased by positive-positive ventilation. Ventilation has its own complications and must not be undertaken lightly. For example, with an asthmatic, it is relatively easy to force air into the lungs, but extremely difficult to get it out again, and a negative pressure applied during expiration only collapses the airways. Such a situation must always be assessed very carefully before ventilation is undertaken.

Artificial ventilation of the lungs is normally carried out by intermittent positive pressure machines, the various types of which are

Care of Respiratory Problems

described in Chapter 9. The machine and circuit appropriate for the patient's condition and size are selected, the ventilator controls given suitable settings, and the circuit connected to the artificial airway. As it is impossible to be sure exactly what the required tidal volume will be in a child, even with the use of nomograms, it is preferable to aim to underventilate at first, and alter the settings to gain adequate chest expansion. Starting with a large volume can lead to the creation of high pressures in the alveoli, perhaps with lung rupture, especially if the patient is breathing against the machine.

Management of a patient on a ventilator

1. *Care of the airway*—as described above.
2. *Sedation* as required. A patient breathing out of time with a ventilator is not being ventilated adequately, and may be harmed. Co-operative patients can be asked to lie still and let the machine do the work, but this is seldom successful with children. Help may be obtained in some children by the use of a sedative, or tranquillizer, such as diazepam.

Careful adjustment of the ventilator setting will also help to keep a patient comfortable. Many people *feel* underventilated even if their $P_a\text{CO}_2$ is normal. This can sometimes be remedied by replacing the catheter mount with a piece of tubing of larger volume, to cause some rebreathing of gases, while the minute volume is then increased without producing hypocarbia, and the patient feels less breathless. It is claimed that some ventilators produce a more even distribution of gas by virtue of their mode of action, and seldom need to be assisted by drugs. Such a machine is the Engström.

However, if there is a strong respiratory drive, producing tachypnoea, as in an infant with bronchiolitis, or if the patient is in status epilepticus, or is just restless and unco-operative, further measures must be taken.

Hypnotics such as chloral hydrate and the barbiturates are seldom successful, and it usually amounts to the choice of a respiratory depressant, such as phenoperidine or other narcotic analgesics, or a muscle relaxant, such as tubocurarine. In many cases, phenoperidine, perhaps combined with droperidol, is quite adequate, but babies, especially those with respiratory infection, are often very resistant to its effects, while on a ventilator. The drug should be given as often as required and not routinely.

If control with a respiratory depressant is unsuccessful, then the patient should be paralysed, to achieve adequate ventilation. However, although conditions are then ideal for ventilation, the patient is competely machine dependent and cannot breathe if the artificial airway should be dislodged. Muscle relaxants are given in dosage calculated from weight, normally intravenously, as often as required, even hourly. Tubocurarine is probably better avoided, as it produces allergic reactions at the site of injection. A similar drug may be used instead—alcuronium or pancuronium.

A patient who is being ventilated with a mixture of oxygen and nitrogen is neither unconscious, nor sedated, and may well have unpleasant memories unless adequately sedated as well as paralysed. Probably diazepam is the drug of choice.

The final excretion of muscle relaxants may be slow, and considerable accumulation may occur in the tissues if the drug is given for several days. Ventilation should be continued until all traces of muscle paralysis have gone, before the patient is allowed to breathe alone. Reversal of the effects of the relaxant with atropine and neostigmine is not advisable, because of the danger of recurarisation after the effects of the neostigmine have diminished.

A patient in status epilepticus should have the fits controlled by reasonable does of antiepileptic drugs if possible, but if these are ineffective, then the patient should be paralysed and artificially ventilated, to allow effective oxygenation, otherwise the brain may be damaged by hypoxia due to hypoventilation.

3. *Care of the unconscious patient.* If a patient is heavily sedated or paralysed, full care must be taken of the skin and pressure areas, of the eyes and mouth, and physiotherapy for the chest and limbs is essential. Attention must be paid to adequate hydration and nutrition.

4. *Monitoring of the ventilator.* These machines require constant supervision, to ensure they are working properly, and to recognise any leaks in the circuit. Observation of the movement of the chest tells the nurse that all is probably well, but hourly recordings of the pressure reached on the manometer, the gas flow and its composition, and the expired minute volume, in older children, should be carried out. The humidifier must be kept filled with water, and any change in the rhythm of ventilation investigated. Arterial or capillary blood is taken for blood gas studies as indicated.

Care of Respiratory Problems

5. *Monitoring of the patient.* Recording of the pulse and respiratory rate, the blood pressure, temperature, and perhaps central venous pressure, is done routinely, as often as is necessary, depending on the condition of the patient. A continuous E.C.G. tracing is shown on an oscilloscope.

Weaning from the ventilator

When the need for artificial ventilation is past, the patient must be encouraged to breathe alone again. All respiratory depressant drugs must be discontinued and time allowed for their elimination. At this stage the patient may become restless, and if the machine is suitable, it is more comfortable for the patient to trigger the onset of inspiration by his own efforts. This is most easily done with the Bird ventilator, but is not a method to be used in infants, partly because of their weakness, partly because they breathe so rapidly. The trigger sensitivity can gradually be decreased, encouraging the patient to greater effort.

With infants, the easiest method of weaning is to allow them to breathe spontaneously for short periods of time. The length of these periods can be gradually increased, making sure the baby does not become too tired. Humidified gases must be breathed at all times. In some babies, spontaneous respiration is accompanied by inspiratory rib recession, especially those with respiratory distress syndrome, pneumonia, and pulmonary venous congestion. This may be partly due to the resistance to breathing given by a long narrow tube, and partly to difficulty in initial lung expansion. This handicap is often greatly improved, and the weaning assisted, by the application of a continuous positive pressure across the airway. Inspiration is assisted, and the extra expiratory effort is well tolerated. The system consists of a supply of humidified oxygen-air mixture, a closed reservoir bag, tubing to and from the patient's airway, the expiratory limb ending under water to a depth equal to the required pressure—usually 5 to 10 cm water.

This circuit can be used alternately with the ventilator to encourage spontaneous respiration, and ultimately the patient will breathe solely with the help of this system. The water level can then be gradually decreased, until the child is breathing alone.

The danger of this circuit is that the expiratory limb may become kinked, in which case a high pressure, exerted by the tense reservoir bag, is placed on the lungs. This complication is easily avoided by the use of suitable tubing, and by making the nurse aware of it. The other problem is that water standing for long periods can readily become infected. The tubing should be changed daily.

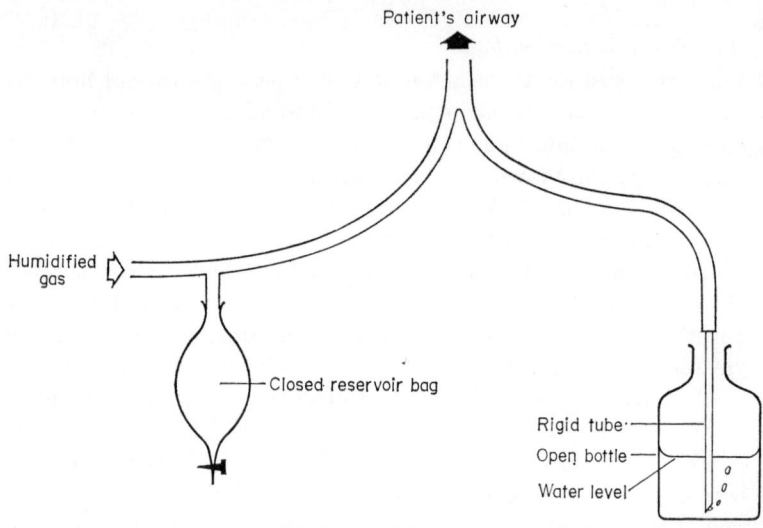

FIG. 12.7 Continuous positive pressure system.

Some babies are weaned by this method, others are better without it. In any case, spontaneous respiration can usually be established. If it cannot, a decision must be made, in consultation, as to whether maintaining life by these artificial means is justified.

Once spontaneous respiration is established, the artificial airway can be removed, and there is no longer a need for intensive care unless other systems require it.

SUMMARY OF MANAGEMENT OF SOME COMMON RESPIRATORY CONDITIONS

Asthma

Aetiology
One or several of allergic, emotional, constitutional and infective factors.

Clinical features
Use of accessory muscles of respiration; poor air entry, expiratory rhonchi; overdistended lungs on X-ray.

Treatment
Bronchodilators—ephedrine, aminophylline, adrenaline.
Aerosols—isoprenaline, orciprenaline.
Antihistamines—e.g. promethazine.
Steroids—if other drugs fail to control spasm.
Antibiotics—if there is an infective element.
Keep well hydrated and oxygenated.

If respiratory failure supervenes—intubation and bronchial lavage with normal saline. As a last resort—artificial ventilation.

Use a volume cycled ventilator for preference, and allow adequate time for expiration. Great care is needed, as lungs may overdistend more, and rupture may occur.

Acid Aspiration Syndrome (Mendelson)

Aetiology
Inhalation of acid gastric contents, giving severe oedema, and spasm of bronchioles. Only a small amount of acid is needed.

Clinical features
Vomiting in unconscious or anaesthetised patient; gastric contents in pharynx; may pass unnoticed; severe tachycardia and tachypnoea may be present; bronchospasm.

Treatment
Immediate intubation, bronchial suction, bronchial lavage with saline. Bronchoscopy if large particles are present. Artificial ventilation if needed; may require high oxygen concentration. X-ray shows patchy opacities but normally no collapse—*do not wait for it* before starting treatment. Steroids—I/V or aerosol hydrocortisone may help to prevent the severe oedema of bronchial tree and alveoli.
Antibiotics.
Physiotherapy.

If treated energetically often no sequelae. In its worst form this condition leads to death from pulmonary oedema and bronchopneumonia.

Acute laryngotracheobronchitis

Aetiology
Virus.

Clinical features
Inspiratory stridor and brassy cough; sternal recession.
Chest X-ray—non-specific.

Treatment
Humid atmosphere—oxygen or air.
Cautious sedation—watch pulse and respiratory rate.

If the child's condition deteriorates, or the pulse or respiratory rate is rising or the $P_a\text{CO}_2$ is rising, or if a combination of these features is present—nasotracheal intubation with small plastic tube for 4–5 days. A course of steroids 24 hours before extubation may be helpful in preventing rebound laryngeal oedema.

Tracheostomy early only if severe laryngeal oedema is present.

Acute epiglottitis

Aetiology
Haemophilus influenzae.

Clinical features
Acute onset, very ill, febrile child; stridor low pitched or absent, epiglottis seen red and swollen in pharynx—beware obstruction; chest X-ray is usually non-specific; organism can be isolated from throat swab and blood culture.

Treatment
Urgent, as sudden death may supervene.
Humid atmosphere.
Antibiotic—chloramphenicol.
Nasotracheal intubation with small plastic tube if obstruction becomes worse. 2–3 days is normally long enough. Rarely, a tube cannot be passed, and tracheostomy would then be necessary.

Pulmonary vascular congestion

Aetiology
Congenital heart lesion, L→R shunts either intra- or extra-cardiac, or congestive cardiac failure.

Clinical features
Signs of the heart lesion, perhaps peripheral oedema and cyanosis; dyspnoea; rib recession; basal pulmonary crepitations; chest X-ray—perihilar opacity, Kerley's lines, pleural fluid.

Treatment
Digoxin and diuretics, fluid restriction.
Surgical correction of lesion if possible, or banding of pulmonary artery, to reduce pulmonary blood flow.
Oxygen by mask or tent.
 If ventilatory failure is present—intubation and artificial ventilation. Volume cycled ventilator is the best, and often necessary, with positive-positive pressure respiratory cycle, long I/E ratio. Tracheostomy if desired. Continuous positive pressure circuit often helps weaning from ventilator.

Respiratory Distress Syndrome of Newborn

Aetiology
Prematurity, ? lack of surfactant in alveoli.

Clinical features
Onset soon after birth, up to the third day, of dyspnoea, rib recession and cyanosis; expiratory grunting; chest X-ray—granular lung fields, 'air bronchogram', translucent patches.

Treatment
High concentration of oxygen, correct any biochemical disturbance. If these measures fail, intubation, and artificial ventilation. Lungs have extremely poor compliance, and a volume-cycled ventilator will be needed, with inspired oxygen concentration just high enough to keep baby pink. Continuous positive pressure circuit may help with weaning. The earlier the onset of the disease, the more severe it is likely to be.

Bronchiolitis

Aetiology
Virus.

Clinical features
Usually infants, starts with a cold, progresses to dyspnoea, severe rib recession, overdistension of lungs, bronchospasm; may be associated with bronchopneumonia; chest X-ray shows flattening of diaphragm and over-distended lungs; cardiac failure may occur.

Treatment
Administer high oxygen by tent usually, attend to hydration. *Very* cautious sedation—watch pulse and respiratory rate. Antispasmodics —e.g. diprophylline.

If ventilatory failure is present—try intubation and bronchial suction. If this is not enough, artificial ventilation will be needed. Volume cycled ventilator preferred, allow time for expiration.

CHAPTER

13

Post-Operative Thoracic Surgical Care

After any operation a rapid return to normal respiratory physiology requires that the functioning lung units must be ventilated, supplied with the appropriate gas mixture, and perfused by desaturated blood in the presence of an alveolar membrane capable of normal diffusion of gases.

Following thoracic or thoraco-abdominal operations the return to a normal physiological state may be hindered by conditions causing interference with the above factors, which are effects of the operation performed.

The essential features of management are:

1. The maintenance of adequate oxygenation; breathing air at normal temperatures often suffices but augmentation by oxygen and/or moisture may be required.
2. The maintenance of a clear airway.
3. The maintenance of normal breathing with a chest wall and diaphragm as actively mobile as possible.
4. The maintenance of an adequate cardiac output.

At rest the whole of the lungs is not usually employed, but blood and air is distributed in a gravitational manner to the most dependent parts (posterior parts if the patient is supine, lung bases if he is sitting up). With the need to increase oxygenation and cardiac output, as in exercise, more of the lungs comes to be used until all areas of both lungs are fully perfused and fully ventilated.

The lung can be considered as being made up of a large number of alveolar units, each consisting of an alveolus receiving air from a respiratory bronchiole and desaturated blood from a branch of a pulmonary arteriole, while oxygenated blood leaves the unit via a pulmonary venule. The normal alveolar unit is ventilated and perfused, and gaseous exchange takes place. If the pre-capillary sphincter to a unit is constricted so that it is not perfused with blood but remains ventilated, this represents an increase of dead space and ineffectual respiratory work is being performed. On the other hand, if bronchiolar obstruction prevents ventilation of the alveolar unit, but perfusion with desaturated blood continues, this blood will not be oxygenated and will pass into the left atrium via the pulmonary veins, so that this will constitute an intra-pulmonary right-to-left shunt.

If, however, an alveolus is neither ventilated nor perfused with blood there will be no increase of respiratory work and no right-to-left shunt, and this can be called a 'silent' unit.

The most common obstacles to oxygen and carbon dioxide transport are:

(a) *Increased right-to-left shunt in the lungs:* There is always *some* shunt present, representing that portion of the cardiac output which does not take part in gaseous exchange but returns to the left heart unoxygenated, and this is mostly the bronchial vein return to the pulmonary veins; this is the *anatomical shunt* which is constant and represents not more than 2 per cent of the cardiac output. To this may be added the variable *capillary shunt* existing when alveolar units are perfused but not ventilated, so that the *total shunt* is a summation of the two varieties. The capillary shunt may be due to conditions causing interference with gaseous diffusion, or uneven distribution of ventilation in relation to perfusion, and if the total shunt is large enough it will produce arterial hypoxaemia and clinical cyanosis when room air is breathed.

(b) *Increased physiological dead space:* Only alveolar ventilation is effective in enabling gaseous exchange to occur, and any inspired gas not taking part in gaseous exchange forms the *total dead space*. Normally the dead space air is that within the air passage as far as the respiratory bronchioles (*anatomical dead space*), but to this must be added the volume of gas used to ventilate non-perfused alveoli (*alveolar dead space*). Non-perfusion of ventilated alveoli thus causes an increase of dead space to tidal volume ratio (V_D/V_T), which may follow haemorrhage, or hypotension, when pulmonary artery flow

Post-Operative Thoracic Surgical Care

under the influence of low pulmonary artery pressure and gravity is preferential to the dependent parts of the lung, leaving some alveoli ventilated but not perfused. A dramatic cause of increased V_D/V_T ratio is, of course, pulmonary embolus.

(c) *Increased respiratory work:* This may be due to increased airway resistance, or to increased elastic resistance against inflation offered by the lung and chest wall (*decreased compliance*).

Airway resistance can be measured as a ratio of pressure gradient over gas flow ($cmH_2O/L/sec$) and since gas flow depends on Poiseuille's equation (Chapters 6 and 7) the airway resistance varies *inversely* as the fourth power of the radius of the air passage. The pressure gradient is the difference in pressure between that at the mouth and in the alveoli.

The distensibility or compliance of the lungs is measured as a ratio of volume change to pressure change ($L/cm\ H_2O$) and may be decreased when there is atelectasis, pulmonary infection, congestion or fibrosis, or a reduction in surfactant.

(d) *Decreased oxygen transport in the blood:* This may be affected by the haemoglobin content of the blood, the inspired oxygen concentration (FI_{O_2}), the volume and distribution of cardiac output, and abnormalities of pulmonary ventilation/perfusion relationships.

Consideration must now be given to the application of the above to the post-operative patient.

GENERAL MANAGEMENT

The patient must be nursed in a position allowing maximal comfort and maximal efficiency of the muscles of respiration. In general, the supine position with perhaps slight anti-Trendelenburg tilt of the cot or bed will provide these requirements, allowing both sides of the chest to expand well with unhindered movement of the rib cage and unimpeded descent of the diaphragm. However, the continuous use of this position may lead to retention of bronchial secretions so that frequent change of position is important to allow proper bronchial drainage of all parts of the lungs, and the patient should be turned in a regular manner, it sometimes being necessary for him to be semi-prone for short periods.

Analgesics to enable the patient to cough effectively without too much discomfort are important, but must not be used to the point of depression of the cough reflex. *Effective* cough enables bronchial secretions to be cleared, and also forces air into the alveoli, maintaining their expansion; ineffective cough may push secretions into the bronchioles and alveoli resulting in collapse/consolidation.

A decision must be taken, based on the patient's general clinical condition and if necessary on the presence of arterial hypoxaemia, as to the need for increasing the oxygen concentration of the inspired gas. It is important for the patient not to breathe *dry* gas as indicated in Chapter 12, so that adequate humidification is important. Supplemental oxygen therapy may be by a suitable disposable face mask if the child will tolerate this, otherwise some variety of oxygen tent must be employed. However, oxygen tents can be frightening to the small child, while observation and access become more difficult, and it is impossible to achieve a very high oxygen concentration. If a tent is employed it should be capable of being cooled (preferably by a refrigeration unit) with a humidifier in the gas input side.

The child's temperature must be measured carefully, and skin recordings are of little value, particularly if the patient is in the wet, cooled atmosphere of an oxygen tent. Recordings should therefore be of the 'core' temperature (that is, the closed mouth, oesophagus, or rectum) but the same site must be selected for all readings as there may be a variation between sites of about 1 °C.

Fluid requirements, blood replacement and nutrition are maintained on the usual lines, blood transfusions being controlled by a careful measurement of loss and, if necessary, central venous pressure recordings. The maintenance of a good cardiac output is very important in order to minimise ventilation/perfusion difficulties.

Acid/base and blood gas determinations are made as often as necessary after operation. Chest radiographs are routinely taken immediately after the operation and thereafter as often as needed.

Pulmonary Atelectasis

This may arise because of bronchial obstruction due to secretions (Active or Absorption collapse), or as a result of pressure on the lung by air, fluid, blood, pus etc. (Passive or comPression collapse). The two varieties require different measures to prevent them and to treat them if they occur, but it is important to appreciate that both types may occur together; for example, a pneumothorax causing partial passive collapse of the lung may be followed by inadequate bronchial drainage, and active collapse.

The distribution may be miliary, lobular, segmental, lobar, or massive involving the whole lung. Early collapse may present dramatically with sudden dyspnoea, high fever, and cyanosis but the onset may be insidious with only a feeling of malaise, reluctance to drink or eat, and a persisting pyrexia. It should be noted that the cyanosis of atelectasis, being due to a right-to-left shunt, does *not* respond to increasing the inspired oxygen concentration. Moreover, if re-expansion does not take place, the cyanosis disappears due to shutting-down of pulmonary perfusion to the collapsed areas and conversion of shunt units to 'silent' units, so that the disappearance of cyanosis does not necessarily mean re-expansion of collapsed lung tissue. *Late* collapse is due to persistence of airless alveoli, although the conditions causing the collapse (e.g. bronchial obstruction) have been relieved. The ultimate effects of atelectasis depend on the extent of associated bacterial invasion and the efficacy of antibiotic therapy.

Prevention and Treatment of Active Collapse

Prevention of active collapse is most likely to be achieved if meticulous attention is paid to pre- and post-operative measures designed to improve ventilation and promote drainage of bronchial secretions. Patients who are old enough to be instructed in postural drainage should be put through the various positions for drainage of the bronchial tree, and shown how to breathe properly (that is, *not* to contract the abdominal muscles when making a forced inspiration) and cough effectively. Drainage of the lower lobes does *not* imply a child hanging over the side of the bed with his weight supported on his hands! It is important for the physiotherapist to be involved in this aspect of patient care at an early stage before operation, but it is of course not possible to do this with the emergency admission, nor in the case of young children and infants. It is recommended that an I.T.U. has its own physiotherapists, who become an integral part of the team. It is desirable that the child should also be introduced to oxygen therapy, whether by mask or tent, and the use of nebulised inhalations. In the case of patients who have chronic respiratory infection it is important to have bacteriological examination of sputum and nose and throat swabs, and a decision must be taken as to the need for pre-operative antibiotic therapy.

If, pre-operatively, pathogenic bacteria are obtained from the respiratory tract, then the patient is given the appropriate antibiotic post-operatively. There is probably no good indication for routine 'prophylactic' antibiotic administration to the non-infected patient undergoing thoraco-abdominal or thoracic surgery, although there may be a need for antibiotic administration in specific instances (for example, intestinal sterilisation in oesophageal reconstructive surgery using colon). The main features of post-operative management are the ensuring of good breathing, a good cough reflex, prevention of drying of bronchial secretions, and adequate analgesia, as already indicated. If gastric distension occurs this should be relieved by the passage of a nasogastric tube otherwise splinting of the diaphragm will impede pulmonary ventilation particularly of the lower lobes.

Post-operative atelectasis occurring despite preventive measures may produce clinical symptoms due to intrapulmonary shunting and infection (arterial hypoxaemia, cyanosis, dyspnoea, tachypnoea, tachycardia and pyrexia), or may cause few symptoms but be detected on a routine post-operative radiograph. *Whether productive of symptoms or not, every effort should be made to achieve re-expansion of early pulmonary collapse due to bronchial obstruction.* Sometimes such collapse is due to the faulty positioning of an endotracheal tube, which occludes a bronchial orifice, and this will respond rapidly to partial withdrawal of the tube. If due to sputum retention, re-aeration of the collapsed segments may follow a period of postural drainage and physiotherapy, but if atelectasis persists an endotracheal tube should be passed under anaesthesia, and endotracheal suction, bronchial lavage and hand inflation of the lungs employed, while in older children bronchoscopic aspiration may be preferable. Material obtained by aspiration is cultured so that any pathogenic bacteria can be isolated and their antibiotic sensitivity determined.

Prevention and Treatment of Passive Collapse

Prevention of passive collapse after operation depends on suitable drainage of pleural fluid, blood, air etc. which would otherwise compress the lung. This does not imply that chest drainage is necessarily required after *all* thoracic operations (for example, following the uneventful ligation of a persistent ductus arteriosus). It is, of course, true that all pleural trauma is followed by some exudation of fluid (just as after an abdominal laparotomy fluid forms in the peritoneal cavity), and indeed the irritation of a pleural drain may provoke exudate, but the pleura is capable of dealing with small effusions quite adequately. If there is any doubt about the possibility of compression of the lung developing post-operatively, then the pleural cavity must be drained at operation. If compression of the lung causes collapse at *any* stage in patient management, the pleural cavity should be aspirated and perhaps drained. The recognition of tension pneumothorax which is life-threatening (particularly if mechanical ventilation of the lungs is being used) is a *clinical diagnosis and must not wait upon radiological confirmation*; the absence of breath sounds, presence of hyperresonance to percussion, and mediastinal shift to the opposite side should be an indication to insert a wide bore needle, mounted on a syringe containing a little sterile water, so that air can be seen to be aspirated; intercostal drainage is then an urgent matter.

An intercostal tube allows fluid and air to drain, and, unless it is inserted into a cavity with rigid walls (for example, chronic empyema) it should be connected to a water seal. A suitable drainage bottle is shown in Fig. 13.1. This consists of a graduated cylinder, closed by a rubber bung through which two metal tubes pass (*not glass* which frequently breaks, injuring the nurse's hands as tubing is attached). Clear plastic tubing leads from one tube under the surface of sterile water added to the bottle to the level 'O', and the other end of this tube is connected by rubber tubing to the intercostal catheter. The latter is preferably of clear polyvinyl chloride and should be a suitable size to pass between the ribs. The rubber connecting tubing must be strong enough not to collapse when suction is applied, but not so rigid that it cannot be 'milked' by the nurse to prevent obstruction by clot. The second tube of the drainage bottle is preferably attached to a vacuum line with the vacuum set to about 10 mm Hg, which promotes drainage from the pleural cavity, encourages lung expansion, and reduces paradoxical breathing. An intercostal drain to an underwater seal normally shows a fluctuating level, this rising on inspiration and therefore constituting paradoxical respiration, which does not greatly matter in a larger child but constitutes a significant volume of wasted inspiration in the infant.

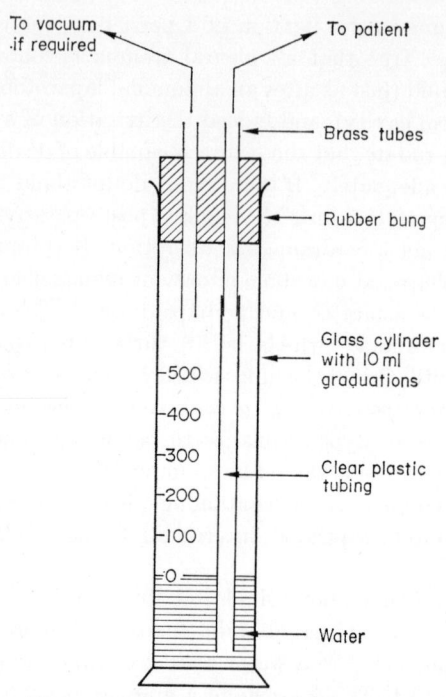

Fig. 13.1 Underwater sealed drainage measuring cylinder.

If a vacuum line is not attached to the second metal tube of the drainage bottle, a mean level is reached of the water rising up the plastic tube, and this represents the negative intrapleural pressure; as indicated, the level rises with inspiration and descends with expiration, the swing being much greater with a violent respiratory effort such as coughing.

It is important that the nature of drainage is recorded (air leaks, blood, pus etc.) and its quantity. The decision to remove intercostal tubes is made after drainage has ceased (after ensuring that the tubes are not blocked) and after radiological confirmation of full lung expansion. If air leak is seen in the drainage bottle, but the lung is fully expanded, one must make sure that air is not sucking in around the drainage tube site.

Intercostal drainage may be required as a matter of life-saving urgency, in which case local anaesthesia for insertion of the tube is not required. A small skin incision is made, a trocar and cannula of suitable size inserted through an intercostal space, the 5th or 6th in the midaxillary line being convenient, and a catheter introduced through the cannula after removing the trocar. It is more convenient and less time-consuming to use a disposable intercostal tube such as the 'Trocath',* which has an intercostal catheter with a radio-opaque sentinel line mounted on its own pointed steel introducer.

If, after instituting intercostal drainage, full lung expansion is not seen on a radiograph but the mediastinum has moved *towards* the side of chest drainage, there is a strong possibility of co-existing active collapse due to bronchial obstruction and the patient may also require bronchoscopy.

Surgical Emphysema

A certain degree of surgical emphysema is almost always found in the subcutaneous tissues in the vicinity of a thoracotomy wound, and indicates that air, present in the pleural cavity, has escaped through the pleural wound into the tissues. This is of no significance.

Gross surgical emphysema can arise in several ways, and can be extremely alarming to the patient and his visitors, as subcutaneous air can spread over the whole body and the eyelids cannot be opened. In a patient with air leak from the lung after a pulmonary resection this state may arise because the intercostal tube is blocked. The condition can also arise after tracheostomy, when violent inspiratory efforts may suck air into the subcutaneous tissues through the cervical incision, and indeed the air may pass into the mediastinum and rupture through the mediastinal pleura in the region of the thymus where the pleura is thinnest, to cause a pneumothorax. Alternatively, surgical emphysema can arise as a result of trapping of air within the lung during expiration, resulting in alveolar rupture and interstitial pulmonary emphysema. The air tracks along the bronchovascular planes to the mediastinum, whence it may rupture into the pleural cavity to cause a pneumothorax, and to the root of the neck where surgical emphysema becomes apparent. Expiratory trapping of air can also cause a pneumothorax directly by rupture of the lung through the visceral pleura directly into the pleural cavity.

* Manufactured by Brunswick Corporation, Worthing, Sussex.

It is particularly important to appreciate that surgical emphysema appearing in the suprasternal notch in a patient whose lungs are mechanically ventilated is an urgent sign that lung rupture has occurred, and that bilateral pneumothoraces may be present, requiring treatment by intercostal underwater sealed drainage.

The treatment of surgical emphysema is the treatment of its cause, and, if necessary, drainage of the pleural cavity. For example, it may occur in obstruction to expiration caused by a foreign body, or obstruction of a tracheostomy tube, and in both instances the obstruction must be relieved. If the subcutaneous air is present as a result of inadequate intercostal drainage then effective drainage should be instituted. There is *no* basis for making incisions in the neck 'to let out the air', a practice formerly carried out because it was believed that air could be present in the superior mediastinum under tension so great that venous return from the head, neck and upper limbs could be impeded.

The Management of Intrathoracic Bleeding

Chest trauma, whether closed or open, may cause bleeding into the pleural cavity or into the lung parenchyma. Bleeding following operation is usually into the pleural cavity, and is obvious if an intercostal drain has been inserted, but concealed haemorrhage should be suspected if there is an unexplained rise in pulse rate, fall in blood pressure, increased respiratory rate and difficulty in ventilating the lung with diminution of the percussion note and absence of breath sounds; this is an indication for chest radiography and diagnostic aspiration of the pleural cavity with institution of intercostal drainage if the presence of blood is confirmed.

The drainage of blood must be measured accurately and blood replacement by transfusion should follow drainage closely, being controlled also by recordings of the systemic arterial pressure and, if necessary, central venous pressure. If drainage ceases, but the lung is not expanded and the chest radiograph shows one side to be opaque, the possibility of clotted haemothorax should be considered provided one is sure that the drainage tubes themselves are not obstructed. Clotted haemothorax is best managed by evacuation at thoracotomy; the presence of clot in the pleural cavity causes malaise and fever, and is a potential risk to the patient because of possible infection, or later by restriction of the lung due to organisation and fibrosis. Fibrinolytic enzymes are slow to clear a clotted haemothorax, and make the patient feel extremely ill in some instances, so that operative removal is preferred to ensure rapid re-expansion of the lung. Moreover, at operation any obvious source of bleeding can be controlled.

Closed trauma sometimes results in a severe contusion of the lung with a diffuse pulmonary opacity on the radiograph and perhaps haemoptysis. There is difficulty in ventilating and perfusing such tissues, and extensive pulmonary contusion has a poor prognosis. Supportive treatment may consist of intermittent positive pressure respiration until the lung has largely cleared.

FURTHER READING

BENDIXEN, H. H., EGBERT, L. D., HEDLEY-WHYTE, J., LAVER, M. B., PONTOPPIDAN, H. (1965) *Respiratory Care*, The C. V. Mosby Company.

CHAPTER

14

Cardiovascular Management

The aim of the surgeon treating congenital cardiovascular disease is to improve the oxygenation of the blood delivered to the tissues, or to diminish the work of the heart needed to supply the blood, or a combination of these.

Broadly speaking, the conditions treated fall into four haemodynamic groups:
1. Simple obstructions in the circulation.
2. Communications between the systemic and pulmonary circulation.
3. Valvular insufficiencies.
4. Varying combinations of the above.

On clinical grounds, we may distinguish non-cyanotic and cyanotic heart disease and these are also divided into groups (Fig. 14.1).

While the above list is by no means complete it illustrates the types of condition found. It is necessary to elaborate on the fundamental physiological derangement in order to determine the treatment necessary and to see how the pre-operative condition and operation affects post-operative management.

Any obstruction in the circulation causes hypertrophy of the pumping chamber proximal to the obstruction with an increase of pressure. Thus in aortic stenosis there is often massive left ventricular hypertrophy with a very high left ventricular pressure. In the case of coarctation of the aorta the high pressure area extends as far as the obstruction which is usually distal to the left subclavian artery, so that there is a high left ventricular pressure and hypertension in

Cardiovascular Management

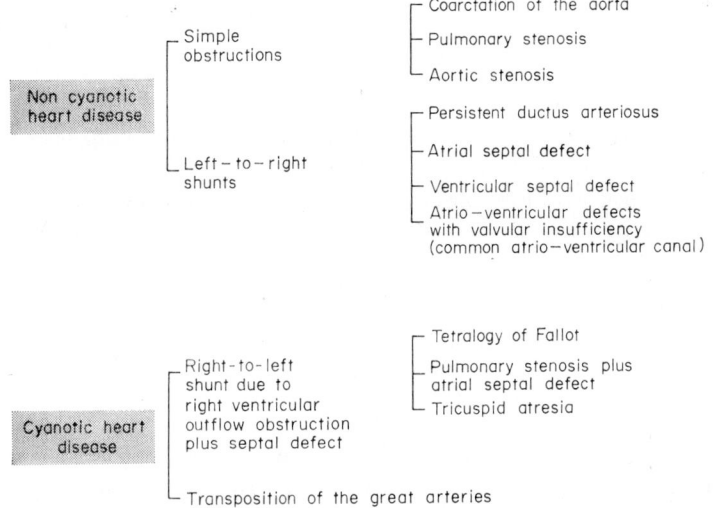

FIG. 14.1 Classification of congenital heart disease.

the arms and carotid arteries. The fundamental haemodynamic difference between aortic stenosis and coarctation lies in the fact that the coronary arteries in aortic stenosis are *distal* to the area of obstruction so that increased left ventricular work is not adequately met by a correspondingly increased coronary artery blood flow. Moreover, in coarctation there is a collateral 'bypass' circulation, a state of affairs which is not possible in valvar obstructions. The effect of left ventricular overwork is eventually ventricular failure, with a lowering of cardiac output. The end diastolic volume and the diastolic pressure rise and ultimately the pulmonary venous pressure rises. When pulmonary venous pressure exceeds 30 mm Hg, fluid begins to leak from the vascular compartment into the interstitial space and alveoli, and the resultant pulmonary oedema hinders gaseous exchange. Pulmonary engorgement with blood, and the accumulation of oedema fluid, both increase the work of breathing (by decreasing pulmonary compliance) leading to dyspnoea, while moist sounds are present on auscultation. In the case of right ventricular failure the systemic venous pressure rises to values of 25–40 mm Hg, the neck veins become distended and the liver enlarges. The elevation of systemic venous pressure is not only due to failure of the right ventricle to pump adequately, but also, in chronic failure, to increase of blood volume. Peripheral venous oedema is first manifested by an increase of body weight, before pitting oedema is found. The production of oedema is a complicated process, involving the retention of water and sodium chloride, so that the total body sodium may be greatly increased, while the serum sodium may be low.

The effect of a left-to-right shunt, at whatever level, is to cause increased pulmonary blood flow with pulmonary engorgement perhaps to the point of causing decreased compliance. Such interference with pulmonary ventilation is more often found in infants, and may lead to a mistaken diagnosis of respiratory infection. The response of the pulmonary arteries to increased blood flow and pressure is either retardation of the normal process of involution, or, if involution has occurred (as in the case of simple atrial septal defects) eventually thickening of the pulmonary artery wall takes place. The object of surgery in treating left-to-right shunts is the prevention or limitation of the anatomical changes of pulmonary hypertension, and the avoidance of the permanent changes of the Eisenmenger state with balancing of the shunt or reversal of the shunt and desaturation of the systemic arterial blood.

The physiological disturbance resulting from cyanotic heart disease is the response of the body to chronic hypoxia, that is, the compensatory over-production of erythrocytes (polycythaemia). While this is necessary in order to increase the oxygen carrying capacity of the blood, it also increases blood viscosity and therefore increases the resistance to flow, resulting in increased cardiac work. Moreover, sluggish flow through smaller vessels may result in intravascular thrombosis, particularly if dehydration has occurred as a result of concurrent illness or climatic conditions. The chronic hypoxia causes severe limitation of effort, and in the case of the Fallot group of patients where the obstruction is in the muscular outflow of the right ventricle and therefore liable to increase at times (infundibular spasm), cyanotic crises can lead to loss of consciousness and possibly convulsions. Such exacerbations of hypoxia will *not* be improved by the administration of oxygen because of poor pulmonary blood flow. The essential difference between cyanotic heart disease of the two main groups is in the lung vascular bed. In the case of the right ventricular obstructions with a right-to-left shunt the lung is poorly vascularised, and may even have evidence of thrombotic occlusion of the smaller vessels, while in uncomplicated transposition of the great arteries there is a hyperdynamic lung circulation with lung plethora and frequently decreased compliance.

The effects of more complicated lesions of the heart, involving combinations of the preceding varieties, will obviously depend on the haemodynamic disturbance resulting from the anatomical malformations, and are beyond the scope of this account.

Treatment of congenital heart disease is essentially a simple concept, the ideal being the restoration of normal physiology by the correction of anatomical defects. Whether full correction is possible or not depends on the severity of the malformation, and whether secondary changes have occurred; thus the irreversible pulmonary hypertension of the Eisenmenger state at the present time implies inoperability.

From the technical point of view, operations on the heart and great vessels fall into two categories:

(a) those which can be carried out at normal body temperature, and without special techniques, e.g. operations for coarctation of the aorta and persistent ductus arteriosus.

(b) Those requiring intracardiac procedures necessitating the use of cardio-pulmonary bypass with or without varying degrees of hypothermia or the use of profound hypothermia.

The necessity for post-operative care in an intensive therapy unit depends on the pre-operative state of the patient, on the complexity of the operation, and on the likelihood of serious post-operative difficulties.

Thus the routine interruption of the persistent ductus arteriosus in a five year old child who has little in the way of symptoms pre-operatively will not require I.T.U. admission, whereas the same operation performed for severe cardiac failure in an infant will certainly be followed by a post-operative period of some anxiety. Whereas the closure of intracardiac left-to-right shunts may be done in children with few symptoms, the complexity of certain procedures and the necessary use of cardio-pulmonary bypass with a possible increased risk of complications requires an I.T.U. post-operative stay which should, however, be conditioned solely by the state of the child, so that, for example, a child who has had an uneventful closure of an atrial or ventricular septal defect could be returned to the ordinary ward on the day after operation.

In order to understand the possible sequelae of cardio-pulmonary bypass it is necessary to give a brief account of the techniques employed.

CARDIO-PULMONARY BYPASS AND PROFOUND HYPOTHERMIA

Circulatory arrest is only safe for about three minutes at normal body temperature, or for about ten minutes at 30°C (so called 'conventional hypothermia'). Operations requiring a longer period of interruption of normal cardiac action are only possible if the action of the heart and lungs is replaced by a machine, or such a degree of cooling is produced that the brain can withstand a longer period of arrest.

Cardio-pulmonary Bypass

Many types of pump oxygenator have been designed, but fundamentally all entail the drainage of venous blood from the superior and inferior vena cava into a chamber where a film of blood is exposed to an oxygen/carbon dioxide mixture (e.g. 97·5 per cent oxygen, 2·5 per cent dioxide). This allows gaseous exchange to occur. Such an oxygenator may consist of rotating steel discs (Kay-Cross), a vertical screen of steel mesh sheets (Mayo-Gibbon), a plastic semi-permeable membrane, or a disposable apparatus such as the Rygg* or Temptrol† oxygenators in which an oxygen/carbon dioxide mixture is allowed to form bubbles in the in-coming venous blood and gaseous exchange takes place at the blood-gas interface of the bubble. The patient must of course be fully heparinized before attaching the machine in order to prevent blood clotting.

The oxygenated blood is then pumped mechanically through a heat exchanger so that the patient's temperature can be modified if necessary, thence through a filter to be returned to the arterial system via a cannula either directly inserted into the aorta or into a large peripheral artery.

During the period of cardio-pulmonary bypass both the heart and lungs are deprived of their normal function. If blood flow to the coronary arteries is interrupted (as may be done intermittently in order to obtain a quiet heart for surgery, and to keep the heart

* Manufactured by Polystan Ltd., Hitchin, Herts.
† Manufactured by Bentley Labs., Santa Ana, California, U.S.A.

Cardiovascular Management

empty by stopping the coronary sinus return) the heart becomes hypoxic; too long periods of hypoxia will affect post-operative function. The lungs still receive blood from the bronchial arteries.

The lungs are usually kept partially inflated during the procedure with periodic full inflation. This is important as otherwise alveolar collapse occurs with possible later difficulty in re-expansion and the production of right-to-left shunts in the lung.

The pump oxygenator itself is usually primed with blood diluted with 5 per cent dextrose or Hartman's solution, the blood being heparinized. Calcium chloride solution is added to the priming solution on account of the high potassium levels in 'bank' blood. Some cardiovascular surgeons use no blood in priming the machine but rely on haemodilution. The admixture of aqueous solutions with the patient's own blood, both from the machine and from pressure monitoring equipment, results in an expansion of the extracellular compartment by fluid which must later be excreted.

At the conclusion of the cardiac procedure the patient is 'weaned' from the pump oxygenator and protamine sulphate is given intravenously to neutralise the heparin. The patient is transfused with blood until the mean left atrial pressure is 20–25 mm Hg, which increases stroke volume and cardiac output to the utmost without overstretching the myocardium and causing cardiac failure.

Biochemical Changes Due to Whole Body Perfusion

If all the body tissues do not receive an adequate amount of fully oxygenated blood they cannot maintain normal aerobic metabolism, so that acid metabolites are formed and a metabolic acidosis results. The acidosis is further increased owing to the dilution of donor blood with acid-citrate-dextrose during its collection. A further possibility is that if a whole blood prime of the pump oxygenator is employed, hypoglycaemic donor blood will cause a release of adrenaline from the recipient's adrenal medulla in order to mobilise liver glycogen to glucose, but muscle glycogen is broken down to lactic acid. This effect is prevented by the use of a dextrose-blood prime.

However adequate the whole body perfusion may be from the pump oxygenator there tends to be a gradual progression of metabolic acidosis proportional to the rate of flow of the perfusate and the duration of perfusion. Even at flow rates near normal resting cardiac output there is *some* metabolic acidosis which is probably related to abnormal regional tissue perfusion resulting from abnormal pressure and flow patterns caused by the non-pulsatile flow of the perfusion.

Progressive increases in serum levels of lactate and pyruvate occur during and immediately after bypass. Lactic acid is the main product of anaerobic glycosis and its production causes a reduction in buffer base. The increased concentration of lactate is a reflection of the decreased tissue Po_2 occurring as a result of impaired tissue perfusion.

If large blood transfusions of acid-citrate-dextrose blood are required after bypass the initial effect will be a lowering of blood pH. However, as the kidney excretes hydrogen ions, and as the citrate is metabolised to bicarbonate by the liver, a metabolic alkalosis usually results, with standard bicarbonate values perhaps in the region of 35 mEq/L.

The catecholamine levels in blood increase during perfusion, with usually an increase of blood glucose, while the plasma concentration of 17-hydroxycorticosteroids increases and lasts after operation until the period of stress ends.

It has been found that children utilize fat for energy throughout bypass operations, even in the presence of high blood sugar levels. The mobilization of glucose causes an increase of serum insulin towards the end of perfusion, but after operation despite reduced intake of glucose the blood level remains fairly normal, with a possibly decreased secretion of insulin. The release of fatty acids during operation leads to a high level of circulating ketone bodies post-operatively, and the findings resemble those of starvation and stress with some insulin insensitivity. This may have important consequences on the body's handling of potassium.

Haematological Changes Associated with Extracorporeal Circulation

Defective blood coagulation following cardio-pulmonary bypass may be a result of one or a combination of the following: a decrease of ionized calcium; increased plasma citrate; deficiency of platelets; consumption of fibrinogen and possibly other coagulation factors (V & VIII); excessive fibrinolysis; incompatible transfusion; heparin rebound; hypothermia or massive blood transfusion itself.

With increasing experience of open heart surgery most units have found that post-operative bleeding problems have become less common. However careful the operative technique may be, the passage of blood through the pump oxygenator with its resulting exposure to foreign surfaces, inevitably leads to loss of formed elements and plasma proteins, while the trauma to which the red cells are exposed causes some fragmentation with an increase of free plasma haemoglobin. The occasional severe post-operative bleeding problem requires the help of the haematological laboratory; the usual causes of such haemorrhage are platelet deficiency, inadequate protamine dosage so that the patient is still partially heparinized, and bleeding from inadequate surgical haemostasis.

It should be noted that certain patients with cyanotic heart disease may have a predisposition to a haemorrhagic diathesis due to accelerated utilisation of clotting factors or alternatively to a high level of circulating fibrinolysins. It has been suggested that this state can be improved before operation by administration of either heparin or ϵ-aminocaproic acid, respectively.

Continued bleeding following bypass may give rise to a vicious circle in that the continued transfusion of blood, while adequately maintaining blood volume, may lead to a progressive further reduction in platelet count since blood which is more than a day old will contain virtually no viable platelets. In addition, massive transfusion will lead to biochemical disturbances.

In the event of excessive continuing haemorrhage following bypass the following tests are indicated:

1. Platelet count: when less than 50,000/cu mm this will contribute significantly to further bleeding and fresh whole blood (or platelet rich plasma or platelet concentrates) should be given.
2. Thrombin time: when prolonged this may indicate excessive residual heparin, fibrinogen depletion due to defibrination or the presence of a fibrinolysin. These can be differentiated in the laboratory by carrying out the appropriate tests in the presence and absence of protamine sulphate and fibrinolytic blockers.

Profound Hypothermia

This implies a reduction of *brain* temperature, as estimated by naso-pharyngeal recordings, to 10°C–15°C. The oesophageal temperature falls rapidly and is usually lower than the naso-pharyngeal, while skeletal muscle temperatures are higher.

Profound hypothermia can be produced by using the heat exchanger of a pump oxygenator to cool the patient, or alternatively the Drew technique in which right and left pumps are employed, the right being used to pump right atrial blood into the pulmonary artery, while the left pumps left atrial blood through a heat exchanger and into the systemic arteries. At the required temperature the pumps are stopped and the intracardiac operation performed. Rewarming is then carried out without exceeding a 10°C difference between the temperature of blood leaving the heat exchanger and the naso-pharyngeal temperature.

Complications of Profound Hypothermia

Children are particularly prone to cold injury, and if an inefficient heat exchanger is employed so that the brain is perfused at normal body temperature with very cold blood, or after circulatory arrest with blood above normal body temperature, or both of these, cerebral damage can result. In addition, if small children and infants have been cooled and are allowed to overheat on rewarming, a state of hyperpyrexia can result due to instability of the temperature regulating mechanism in the hypothalamus, with convulsions and cardiovascular collapse.

The other complications are those which may be associated with the pump oxygenator procedure.

MAINTENANCE OF ADEQUATE CARDIAC OUTPUT

Cardiac output may be low after operation as a result of:
1. Low circulating blood volume
2. Cardiac tamponade
3. Inadequate contractility of the myocardium and cardiac failure
4. Hypoxaemia
5. Acidosis (metabolic or respiratory)
6. Electrolyte disturbances
7. Inadequate heart rate, e.g. atrioventricular block
8. Cardiac arrhythmias
9. 'Shock' and the 'low cardiac output syndrome'

The type and frequency of patient monitoring necessary in addition to the usual ward recordings of temperature, pulse, respiratory rate and blood pressure will depend on the patient's condition. In most instances systemic arterial pressure and central venous pressure will be measured via indwelling cannulae, this having the advantage that the cannulae are available for the withdrawal of arterial or venous samples for blood gas and biochemical investigations. The acid/base state and Po_2 are assessed as often as required, initially frequently (perhaps every 2 hours), this being particularly necessary in the early stages of establishing a patient on assisted ventilation.

The signs of a low circulating blood volume are a poorly palpable thready pulse, with a low arterial pressure, low central venous pressure, and peripheral vasoconstriction. The commonest cause in post-operative cardiac surgical patients is inadequate blood replacement, so that accurate measurement of blood loss occurring through drainage tubes, with prevention of clotting or pooling of blood in the pericardium, pleural cavity and mediastinum, is extremely important. Blood replacement therapy should follow drainage very closely. Blood loss causes a decreased blood volume with a lowering of the filling pressure, a decreased end diastolic volume and therefore a decreased stroke volume so lowering output. Reduced tissue perfusion and hypoxia will cause a metabolic acidosis, in itself contributory to impaired cardiac function. Impaired renal blood flow accentuates the acidosis as the kidney inadequately excretes hydrogen ions. Unless adequately treated, hypovolaemic lowering of cardiac output can cause the patient to enter the vicious circle of 'shock' as shown in Fig. 14.2.

Blood replacement must be carefully controlled by recording of systemic arterial and central venous pressure every fifteen minutes. In general, transfusion is safe provided the central venous pressure does not rise above the upper limit of normal. Raising the atrial and end diastolic ventricular pressures increases the stroke volume and cardiac output, and in many units it is now the practice to record right and left atrial pressures; if the mean pressure in the right atrium is 10 mm Hg, and that in the left is 15 mm Hg, an adequate blood volume and circulation can usually be assumed. A higher than normal atrial pressure may indicate failure of the corresponding ventricle, but it should be noted that some patients (for example, after correction of tetralogy of Fallot) require a high central venous pressure in order to maintain an adequate systemic arterial pressure.

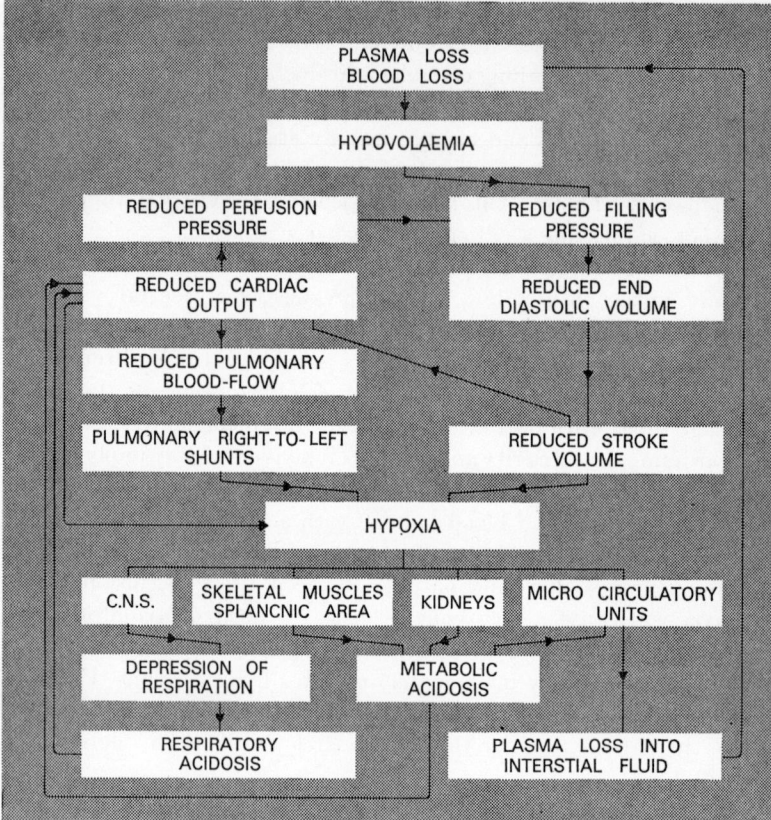

Fig. 14.2 Effects of Hypovolaemia.

Inefficient drainage of blood from the pericardium, and sometimes from the retrosternal space, will cause cardiac tamponade, the compression of the ventricles interfering with diastolic filling so that there is diastolic hypertension on both sides of the heart with systemic and pulmonary venous congestion and reduced cardiac output. The central venous pressure slowly rises, the systemic arterial pressure falls and the heart beat is barely palpable with muted sounds on auscultation. *This obviously cannot be remedied by transfusion* but must be treated by evacuation of the compressing clot. It is important to distinguish low output due to tamponade from that due to a poorly functioning myocardium.

Cardiovascular Management

Inadequate contractility of the myocardium and cardiac failure may be due to the pre-operative state of the patient or may result from post-operative hypoxaemia, acidosis, or electrolyte disturbances such as an impaired calcium/sodium/potassium balance as indicated in Chapter 4. It is important when administering blood to give intravenously 5 ml of 10 per cent calcium gluconate solution for every 500 ml of acid-citrate-dextrose blood transfused. The management of poor cardiac function is primarily that of correcting the cause of the low output, the commonest of these being inadequate maintenance of blood volume and inadequate pulmonary ventilation. Metabolic acidosis occurs in patients who have a continuing low cardiac output and inadequate tissue perfusion. An alkalotic state, on the other hand, may result from metabolism of the citrate in transfused blood, or the addition of sodium bicarbonate or buffer to the pump priming solution. A metabolic alkalosis may have been present before operation if total body potassium level has been reduced by prolonged treatment with diuretics. Reduction of cardiac output due to metabolic acidosis requires measures to improve tissue perfusion and correct the low pH by intravenous sodium bicarbonate as indicated in Chapter 5. In order to avoid giving too great a sodium load, buffers such as THAM (trishydroxymethylaminomethane) may be used, the amount required being calculated as body weight in Kg × base deficit mEq/L in ml of 0·3 M THAM. A further effect of metabolic acidosis is the relaxation of the pre-capillary sphincters of the microcirculatory units, while catecholamine release causes constriction of the post-capillary sphincters, the net result of which is loss of fluid from the vascular compartment into the tissue spaces with a reduction of cardiac output. Moreover acidosis causes renal shut-down so that the kidney can play a decreasingly effective role in correcting the acid/base disturbance. Respiratory acidosis also has a directly depressant effect on cardiac action and renal blood flow.

Interference with cardiac conduction can cause varying degrees of atrioventricular block or a very slow nodal rhythm may be present, both of which can cause a lowering of cardiac output. Complete heart block is particularly serious, and if occurring during operation is managed by the insertion of pacemaker leads into the ventricular muscle and direct electrical pacing of the heart. If heart block occurs in the intensive therapy unit the lowering of cardiac output can be treated immediately by intravenous isoprenaline, and occasionally will prove to be temporary. Continuing heart block must be treated by the insertion of an endocardial pacing catheter via a peripheral vein into the right ventricle, this preferably being done under radiological screening control using an image intensifier. The lowest pacing voltage producing cardiac contraction is selected, and the rate adjusted according to the age and size of the child in order to obtain a good systemic arterial pressure. A careful watch must be kept on the electrocardiogram to detect possible resumption of normal sinus rhythm because interference from the pacemaker then carries the risk of inducing ventricular fibrillation.

Cardiac arrhythmias occurring post-operatively include paroxysmal atrial tachycardia, multiple ventricular premature contractions, ventricular tachycardia and ventricular fibrillation. An arrhythmia may be due to potassium depletion and is then particularly likely to occur if the patient is receiving digitalis. Disturbances of rhythm due to acid/base or electrolyte imbalance respond to the appropriate correction, but if the cause is unknown corrective measures include synchronised defibrillation for atrial tachycardia (inadvisable in the digitalised patient for fear of inducing ventricular fibrillation), and direct current counter shock for ventricular fibrillation. A tendency to repeated episodes of arrhythmia, particularly in the digitalised patient, is treated by intravenous phenytoin, the dose being 1·5 mg/Kg intravenously, repeated in an hour if necessary, and followed by the same dose orally or intravenously, every six hours. If the arrhythmia does not respond to this, intravenous lignocaine is employed, the loading dose being 1–2 mg/Kg body weight, and the intravenous infusion containing 1 gm of lignocaine per 200 ml being continued at a rate of 20–50 μg/Kg/min.

If no apparently correctable causes of low cardiac output are present it is necessary to try to improve output by improving myocardial contractility. It is preferable to begin such supportive treatment at an early stage, and unless contraindications are present, or the patient is already adequately digitalised, digoxin is given intravenously. The total digitalising dose is 0·9 mg/M^2 of body surface, and of this dose two thirds is given *slowly* intravenously, with electrocardiographic control, followed by one sixth after six hours and the remaining one sixth after a further six hours. Care must be taken to ensure that there is an adequate serum potassium level.

Very urgent treatment of low output requires the intravenous use of a catecholamine. Because of its predominantly alpha-adrenergic receptor stimulation nor-adrenaline is not employed, while adrenaline has variable vasoconstricting effects so that its use may be followed by metabolic acidosis. Both of these catecholamines have the side effect of lowering renal perfusion. Isoprenaline, having entirely beta-adrenergic effects, is the drug of choice, and in addition to inotropic and chronotropic effects on the heart dilates all vascular beds including that of the kidney. Care must be taken to maintain an adequate circulating blood volume in view of the vasodilatation. A suitable concentration is 0·6–0·8 mg/250 ml of transfusion solution, the rate being adjusted to maintain the systemic arterial pressure at 90–100 mm Hg systolic.

Some patients after major cardiac reconstructive operations develop a state of 'shock' or the 'low cardiac output syndrome' in which a vicious circle is set up of high central venous pressure, low cardiac output with a low mean systemic arterial pressure, profound vasoconstriction with cold extremities, oliguria or anuria, and metabolic acidosis. Such a state was formerly called 'irreversible shock' but perhaps the term refractory hypotension is more meaningful. A logical attack on this condition will include the use of an intravenous infusion of isoprenaline to improve cardiac output, with alpha-adrenergic blockade by phenoxybenzamine (1 mg/Kg of body weight). *This requires caution* and very careful monitoring of systemic arterial and central venous pressures is necessary, as the circulating blood volume will require expansion to cope with the vasodilatation. Administration of sodium bicarbonate or THAM will also be required to restore the low pH. In some patients an improvement of cardiac output and peripheral vasodilatation will result from intravenous injection of a *large* dose of steroid given as a 'bolus' (see appendix).

OTHER CARDIOVASCULAR DISTURBANCES

Certain other aspects of management of cardiovascular operations in childhood require mention, for example, patients who have had a persistent ductus arteriosus interrupted may develop a reflex tachycardia lasting for several hours after operation, but this does *not* necessarily indicate concealed haemorrhage or the need for digitalisation. Similarly, some patients who have had the blood flow to the distal aorta suddenly increased after operation for a coarctation have a rebound hypertension exceeding the pre-operative level. This is of extreme importance in that the blood vessels now receiving blood at increased flow and pressure react by constriction, and necrotizing arteritis can result, which is particularly disastrous in the mesenteric vessels. A systolic pressure consistently raised above 200 mm Hg, particularly if associated with abdominal pain, is ominous, and is an indication for the use of a hypotensive agent such as reserpine.

It has already been stated that the central venous pressure is required to be higher than normal after correction of tetralogy of Fallot in some patients, in order to maintain a good cardiac output. Other procedures may cause some interference with normal systemic venous return (for example, the reconstruction of the atrial septum in the Mustard operation for transposition of the great arteries, or the superior vena cava–right pulmonary artery anastamosis of Glenn for tricuspid atresia). In such instances the high venous pressure causes cerebral and facial venous congestion with facial (and possible cerebral) oedema, and posture is extremely important in management, the child being sat up to an angle of 45 degrees.

Palliative procedures for patients with right ventricular obstruction and septal defects, in which closed infundibular resection is done, are sometimes followed by a state of severe cyanosis and profound hypoxia, with restlessness, loss of consciousness or convulsions. Such a condition unless due to pulmonary causes must be due to increased right-to-left shunting in the heart, attributable to infundibular spasm, and this can be treated by beta-adrenergic blockade using propranolol (which does, however, have the disadvantage of leaving the coronary arteries unprotected from the alpha-stimulating effects of circulating catecholamines).

In patients who have been polycythaemic before operation, maintenance of blood volume may not necessarily be by blood transfusion. For example, after an aorto-pulmonary shunt as a palliative procedure for cyanotic heart disease, intravenous plasma or plasma substitute such as low molecular weight dextrans may be preferable. It should be borne in mind however that the dextran solutions all interfere with blood coagulation, which may be

THE LUNGS AND CARDIAC SURGERY

Some interference with respiratory function is found in all patients after surgery, and this may involve decreased oxygenation as well as impaired ventilation. It is obvious that the patient who has had congested lungs prior to operation due to a left-to-right shunt, or who develops pulmonary venous congestion after operation, will have 'stiff' lungs which he has difficulty in ventilating. Less obvious is the reason for some degree of arterial desaturation lasting for several days after operation, which is due to perfusion of non-ventilated alveoli with a resulting right-to-left shunt in the lungs. Such areas of pulmonary collapse are not usually evident in chest radiograph and are referred to as miliary atelectasis.

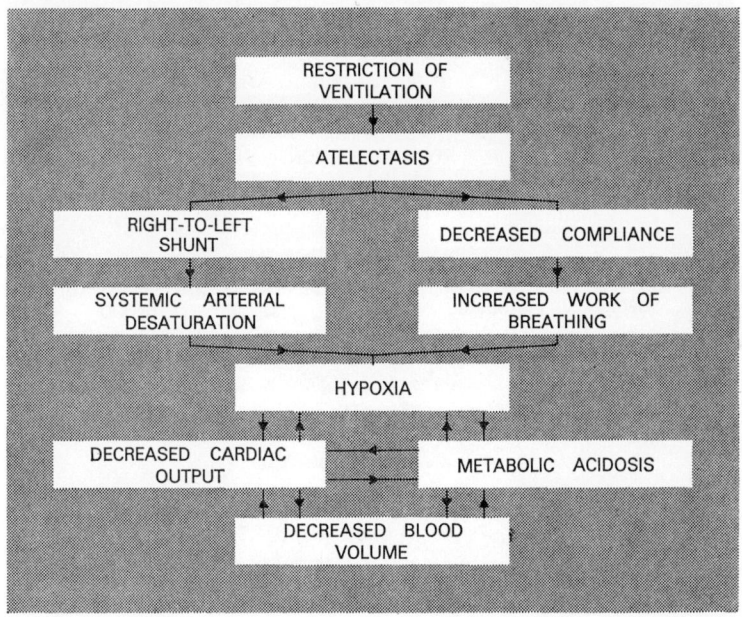

FIG. 14.3 Effect of Restriction of Ventilation on Cardiac Function.

The factors causing restriction of ventilation are pain, compression of the lung by air or fluid (e.g. haemothorax) and pulmonary conditions secondary to cardiac lesions. Restriction of breathing leads to atelectasis, and this has the effect of producing a right-to-left shunt, and also of decreasing lung compliance. Both of these cause hypoxaemia, with depression of cardiac function, poor tissue perfusion and the production of a metabolic acidosis leading to a reduction of blood volume by fluid loss into the extravascular compartment as already described. The changes are illustrated in Fig. 14.3.

Alveolar hypoventilation in the post-operative period causes inadequate gaseous exchange with an increased $P_a{co_2}$, and this respiratory acidosis reduces cardiac output. Depression of the rate and depth of ventilation is caused by pain, persistence of the effects of anaesthesia or premedication, or the injudicious use of analgesics post-operatively. The effects are summarised in Fig. 14.4.

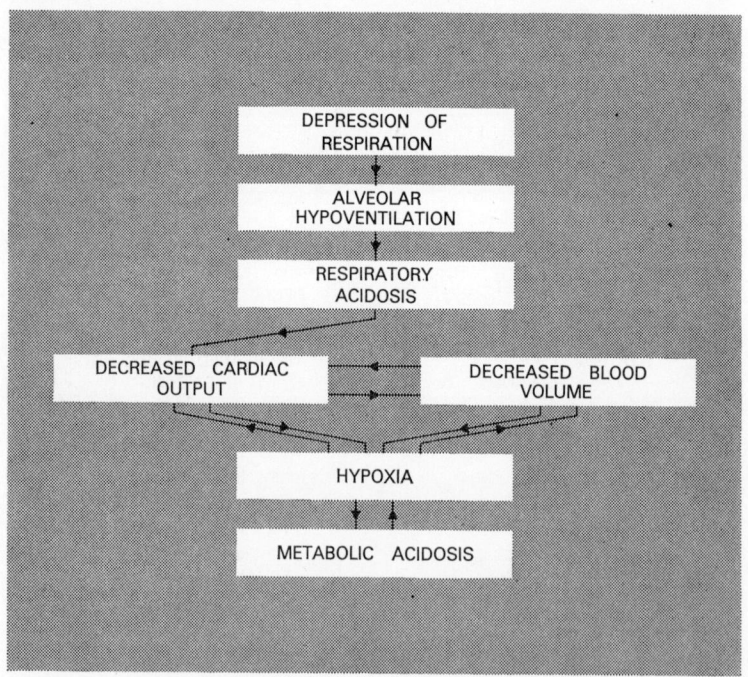

FIG. 14.4 Effect of Depression of Ventilation on Cardiac Function.

OTHER FEATURES OF CARDIOVASCULAR MANAGEMENT

Fluid and electrolyte balance are extremely important in cardiac surgical patients, and no hard and fast rules can be given. On the one hand there is the need to avoid giving a patient too much water and sodium chloride, particularly if cardiac failure has been present before operation or some degree of failure is present post-operatively; on the other hand, too great a degree of dehydration is inadvisable both from the point of view of renal function, and particularly in polycythaemic patients in whom there is a real risk of intravascular thrombosis. As a general rule, in cardio-pulmonary bypass surgery fluid is given on the day of operation to the total of 800 ml/M^2 of body surface/24 hours including that given during the bypass procedure, and during the next 24 hours the same volume is given together with a volume equal to the quantity of urine passed and an amount compensating for extrarenal losses (e.g. gastric aspirate). The composition of the basic fluid will depend on acid/base and electrolyte determinations, and may consist of only 5 per cent dextrose, or 4·3 per cent dextrose and 0·18 per cent sodium chloride. Intravenous potassium administration, unless the serum level is very low, is preferably withheld until urine secretion is well established.

The urine output after operation may be low as a result of poor renal perfusion during operation. Oliguria may result from continued low cardiac output, from metabolic and renal 'shut down', from the alpha-adrenergic receptor stimulation by catecholamines, or simply because not enough fluid has been given. The accurate measurement of the volume of urine passed, by catheter, and its specific gravity, is of fundamental importance in management.

The patient's cerebral state also requires careful assessment after operation. Restlessness despite moderate analgesia is usually due to hypoxia, the cause of which should be sought and corrected. The failure to regain consciousness after operation may be due to cerebral air embolism in the case of open heart surgery, when hypothalamic disturbance can result in hyperpyrexia; the unconscious state is usually accompanied by a bizarre neurological picture, varying from a minor degree of pyramidal tract lesion and hemiplegia at one end of the spectrum to spastic decerebrate rigidity at the other. Unconsciousness may be accompanied by convulsions, and other factors may be 'sludging' of the red cells in the cerebral circulation, or cerebral thrombosis. The management of the unconscious state is described in Chapter 17.

The patient's temperature is important, and the ambient temperature in the case of infants is critical, since they are very dependent on environmental conditions. The pyrexia consequent on trauma is expected in the cardiac patient as in any other, but greatly raised temperatures are to be avoided owing to the increased metabolic rate and therefore increased need for oxygen. An increased temperature is sometimes associated with peripheral vasoconstriction which prevents loss of heat from the body 'core'; this can be remedied by promoting vasodilatation, to allow heat to be conducted to the periphery. On the other hand, excessive heat loss with production of subnormal temperatures results in peripheral vasoconstriction in an attempt to conserve body heat, with metabolic acidosis as the consequence.

CHAPTER
15

Acute Renal Failure

Acute renal failure may be defined as an abrupt cessation of the kidneys' ability to maintain regulation of the volume and composition of the body fluids. The resulting biochemical disturbances worsen from day to day, rather than over a period of months or years as in chronic renal failure, and therefore demand urgent treatment.

Normal renal function requires not only intact nephrons, but also an adequate blood supply to perfuse them, and an unobstructed outlet for the urine formed. It is therefore essential to recognise the existence of what are conventionally termed *pre-renal* and *post-renal* factors, as well as the parenchymal disorders themselves.

PRE-RENAL FAILURE

The renal blood flow will be reduced whenever there is a fall of circulating blood volume, blood pressure or cardiac output. Some of the more important causes in childhood are shown in Table 15.1.

Table 15.1 The main causes of pre-renal failure in infancy and childhood.

1. *Burns*—more than 15 per cent body surface area
2. *Major injury*
3. *Massive haemorrhage*
4. *Anaesthesia and operative surgery*
5. *Gastroenteritis*—severe dehydration
6. *Septicaemia*—especially gram-negative
7. *Congestive cardiac failure*
8. *Nephrotic syndrome*—severe hypoalbuminaemia
9. *Anaphylactic shock*—e.g. bee stings, penicillin etc.

Most of the blood entering the kidney is distributed to the cortex, and the main initial effect of circulatory insufficiency is a fall of glomerular filtration rate (GFR) resulting from defective glomerular perfusion. Trauma, whether accidental or surgically induced, always causes a temporary fall of GFR, accompanied by increased secretion of the antidiuretic hormone (ADH), and this results in oliguria with concentrated urine, provided that the GFR is not reduced by more than about one third. Transient oliguria and a modest rise of blood urea level frequently follow such events, and may be regarded as physiological. A more severe fall of GFR, however, impairs the kidney's concentrating ability despite normal ADH secretion. Thus the urinary concentration provides a crude but nonetheless useful means of distinguishing physiological oliguria from pre-renal failure. Provided that the ischaemia is of short duration the renal cortex will escape damage, or at most there may be patchy, focal tubular necrosis. With intact proximal tubules, sodium reabsorption remains unimpaired, yielding a low urinary sodium concentration, but with the development of substantial tubular necrosis, reabsorption diminishes and the urinary concentration rises.

The list of causes of pre-renal failure given in Table 15.1 is not exhaustive and the relative frequency will vary according to the type of clinical service. Uniform depression of both GFR and effective renal plasma flow has been found in children with burns involving 15 per cent or more of body surface area. Where the burns cover more than 40 per cent of surface area these changes become more severe and azotaemia invariably develops, many patients progressing to irreversible renal failure. Post-operative hypotensive and hypovolaemic episodes are nowadays swiftly recognised and corrected, but profound falls of renal blood flow are sometimes experienced after major cardiothoracic surgery. In gastroenteritis, fluid loss into the intestine precedes diarrhoea and vomiting, and hypovolaemic shock may develop rapidly. Profound shock may also develop with alarming rapidity when gram-negative bacteraemia complicates such illnesses as meningococcal meningitis or peritonitis. A slight fall of GFR necessarily follows the reduced cardiac output of cardiac failure, but usually only physiological oliguria and a mild rise of blood urea level results. In the nephrotic syndrome the plasma volume is diminished owing to the lowering of osmotic pressure caused by leakage of proteins—especially albumin—into the urine. There is invariably

Acute Renal Failure

oliguria, and often a modest rise of blood urea level, during the oedematous stage, but rarely the circulating plasma volume may be so low as to result in a substantial fall of GFR, with pre-renal failure. Anaphylactic reactions are uncommon, and death from profound shock may occur before the renal effects of circulatory failure have time to become manifest.

In several of the conditions mentioned, a hypercatabolic state also exists, creating a bigger load of nitrogenous waste for the kidneys to excrete. This is particularly so in patients with severe infections, extensive burns, and following major surgery or accidental trauma. It adds considerably to the problems of patients with renal insufficiency, while in the presence of normal renal function it may lead the unwary medical attendant to diagnose renal failure.

POST-RENAL FAILURE

Sudden and complete obstruction of the urinary tract is an uncommon event in childhood, and its main importance is in the differential diagnosis from true renal failure. Anuria due to urethral compression may result from faecal impaction with unrecognised constipation. Total obstruction in boys may result from urinary tract infection superimposed upon posterior urethral valves.

In order to cause anuria, obstruction at a level higher than the bladder must, of course, be bilateral, unless there is a congenitally absent or non-functioning kidney on one side. Recognition of the potential toxicity of sulphonamides in dehydrated children has virtually abolished crystallisation as a cause of obstruction.

RENAL PARENCHYMAL FAILURE

In true renal failure there is no response to the correction of hypotension or hypovolaemia, when present, or to the administration of osmotic diuretics. Both circulatory insufficiency and total obstruction may lead to renal parenchymal failure if prolonged. Bilateral, obstructive lesions should rarely escape diagnosis, and previously healthy kidneys recover surprisingly well following the relief of acute obstruction of short duration. Reference to Table 15.2 shows that there are two varieties of acute tubular necrosis (ATN)—*ischaemic* and *nephrotoxic*. In the ischaemic type the necrosis involves the tubular basement membrane as well as the epithelial cells, leading to occasional ruptures with leakage of tubular contents into the interstitial tissue. These changes are generally of focal distribution, whereas in the nephrotoxic lesion cellular necrosis is more widespread but the basement membrane remains intact.

Table 15.2 Some causes of acute tubular necrosis (ATN) in infancy and childhood.

---
1. *Ischaemic*—as listed in Table 15.1
2. *Nephrotoxic*
   (a) Massive intravascular haemolysis—e.g. 'blackwater fever', mismatched blood transfusion.
   (b) Ingested poisons—e.g., chlorinated hydrocarbons used as organic solvents, concentrated phenolic antiseptics, ethylene glycol (antifreeze), methyl alcohol.
   (c) Medically administered substances—e.g. antibiotics, (kanamycin, colomycin, polymyxin), heavy metals (especially mercury), contrast media injected i/v in high concentration.
   (d) Miscellaneous—e.g. snake venom, carbon monoxide, electric shock.

The mechanism of oliguria in ATN is poorly understood. The concept of renal vasoconstriction is attractive in that it might be considered as a compensatory mechanism for circulatory collapse, to protect more immediately vital organs such as the brain, heart and lungs. It is now believed, however, that reasonable renal blood flow is re-established after the initial insult. Diversion of blood from cortical glomeruli into the medulla, via the juxta-medullary glomeruli, might explain continuing oliguria despite an adequate renal blood flow. This is supported by the typical post mortem appearance of cortical pallor and medullary congestion in patients dying during the oliguric phase of ATN. Interstitial oedema may also contribute to the production of oliguria, as a rise of intra-renal pressure would oppose both renal artery perfusion and glomerular filtration. Obstruction of tubules by necrotic cellular debris and casts may initially enhance this effect. The brisk diuresis which heralds recovery could also be explained by the disappearance of interstitial oedema.

Ischaemic ATN is commoner than the nephrotoxic type in childhood. Mismatched blood transfusion is a rare accident, but massive haemoglobinuria occurs from time to time where malignant tertian malaria is prevalent. The nephrotoxicity of the drugs mentioned in

Acute Renal Failure

Table 15.2 is widely known and they are not commonly used, while adverse reactions to contrast media are rare.

The causes of acute renal failure other than ATN are shown in Table 15.3.

Table 15.3 Causes of acute renal parenchymal failure other than ATN in infancy and childhood.

1. *Glomerular—vascular disease*
    (a) Acute post-streptococcal glomerulonephritis
    (b) Rapidly progressive glomerulonephritis (including Schönlein-Henoch purpura)
    (c) Lupus nephritis
    (d) Polyarteritis nodosa
    (e) Haemolytic-uraemic syndrome
2. *Bilateral renal infarction*
    (a) Renal venous thrombosis
    (b) Renal arterial occlusion
3. *Symmetrical cortical necrosis*
4. *Acute on chronic renal failure*

An onset of glomerulonephritis with acute renal failure is ominous because of its association with the rapidly progressive form, in which large epithelial crescents obliterate the filtration space between the glomerular tufts and Bowman's capsules in more than 80 per cent of glomeruli. Sometimes, however, there is post-streptococcal glomerulonephritis of no more than average severity, from which complete recovery is possible if the child can be kept alive until a diuresis occurs. Rapidly progressive glomerulonephritis is rare in childhood, and most cases are associated with Schönlein-Henoch purpura. The commonest intrinsic cause of renal failure in childhood is the haemolytic-uraemic syndrome, which affects predominantly children aged 6 months–2 years, and the acute renal failure is caused by massive blood coagulation within the glomerular capillary loops. The mechanism of renal failure in this group of disorders is clear cut; occlusion of the glomerular capillaries by proliferating cells or blood clot, or of the afferent arterioles themselves by fibrinoid deposits, prevents glomerular filtration, and tubular changes are mainly secondary.

Renal infarction in childhood is virtually confined to venous thrombosis, which affects mainly neonates who become dehydrated. Renal failure only occurs when both kidneys are extensively infarcted. Patchy, focal renal cortical necrosis is probably a fairly common event with little clinical significance in children with circulatory failure, but the symmetrical form in which ischaemic necrosis involves all the cortical structures of both kidneys and is uniformly fatal, is a rare complication, usually of severe gastroenteritis. Acute renal failure is sometimes the first evidence of serious underlying kidney disease, such as bilateral renal hypoplasia or chronic pyelonephritis.

METABOLIC DISTURBANCES

Azotaemia

Normal metabolic processes, including the breakdown of dietary protein, lead to the production of non-protein nitrogen, mainly in the form of urea, creatinine and uric acid, which accumulate in the body fluids if the kidneys are unable to excrete them. Renal function is more closely reflected by plasma creatinine levels than by those of urea, which are considerably influenced by pre-renal factors. A modest rise of blood urea accompanies dehydration or tissue trauma even in the presence of normal renal function, but, when there is renal failure in addition, conditions such as severe burns or septicaemia substantially increase the load of urea to be excreted, resulting in a rapid rise of plasma level.

Sodium and Water Imbalance

In the absence of adequate glomerular filtration the responses to aldosterone and ADH, which are mainly responsible for regulating the volume and osmolality of the extracellular fluid, break down, with the result that both sodium and water are retained. The water content is increased to a barely significant degree by metabolism. However, a continuing fluid intake leads to progressive dilution of plasma and extracellular fluid, with consequent hyponatraemia.

Hyperkalaemia

In health, the dietary potassium intake is balanced by the output and the renal regulatory mechanism maintains a low plasma concentration. In renal failure, potassium excretion is severely impaired and, even if it is excluded from the diet, plasma levels will continue to rise slowly owing to the release from cells which accompanies tissue metabolism. When the patient is also severely acidotic or in a hypercatabolic state the plasma level may rise rapidly, and there is considerable risk of cardiac arrest from potassium intoxication.

Acidosis

In normal health the unwanted excess of hydrogen ions produced by cellular metabolism and dietary protein breakdown are normally excreted by the kidneys, while the bicarbonate formed in the tubular cells is returned to the extracellular fluid. In acute renal failure the accumulation of hydrogen ions lowers the blood pH and also its concentration of bicarbonate, which is used in buffering, while, in an attempt to compensate for the acidosis, the P_{CO_2} is reduced by hyperpnoea.

Anaemia

The kidney plays an undefined part in erythropoiesis, and in acute renal failure there is usually normochromic anaemia from decreased erythrocyte production, which may be enhanced by haemolysis. This is usually more severe in the presence of sepsis, and in the case of extensive burns or trauma the picture may be complicated by blood loss.

Bleeding Tendency

Although most patients maintain normal platelet counts, a qualitative defect of platelet function, resulting in an increased bleeding time, is frequently found.

CLINICAL MANIFESTATIONS

The usual presenting symptom of acute renal failure is oliguria, although occasionally dilute urine may be passed in normal quantities, despite the presence of ischaemic ATN and all the metabolic consequences of renal failure. The lower limit of normal urine output is not well defined, especially in young children, but an output of less than 200 ml/M^2/24 hours is abnormally low in the presence of an adequate blood circulation.

The role of azotaemia as a cause of symptoms is not clear. The early symptoms of lassitude, anorexia, nausea and vomiting, followed by stomatitis, diarrhoea, gastrointestinal bleeding, drowsiness and twitching, and ultimately progressing to coma and convulsions, are related to the combination of biochemical disturbances outlined above rather than to the uraemia alone, and probably also to the rapidity with which they develop.

The water and sodium retention may cause slight peri-orbital oedema. A continuing intake of hypotonic fluids, orally or intravenously, will cause progressive dilutional hyponatraemia and, if unchecked, can lead to water intoxication, with convulsions. Failure to recognise the nature of the hyponatraemia, coupled with misguided attempts to correct it with isotonic saline, will exacerbate peripheral oedema and may also lead to hypertension, pulmonary oedema and cardiac failure. The main clinical effect of acidosis is the deep, sighing respiration by means of which carbon dioxide is removed from the blood.

Hypertension may or may not be present, depending upon the cause of renal failure and the degree of sodium overload. Pericarditis may develop in advanced uraemia, and is suggested by a feeling of discomfort in the chest, or substernal pain. Undoubtedly the most serious threat to cardiac action is that from hyperkalaemia. With serum potassium levels rising above 8 mEq/L, cardiac arrhythmias are likely to develop and there is a risk of cardiac arrest. The effects of hyperkalaemia are aggravated by acidosis, and also by hypocalcaemia, which may be present in children suffering from acute on chronic renal failure. An extra strain may be imposed on the heart by severe anaemia. Anaemia also accounts for the pallor which is characteristic of acute renal failure, and may be exacerbated by bleeding from the gastrointestinal tract as well as from incisions and injection sites.

DIAGNOSIS

The diagnosis of renal failure demands as much skill as its treatment. The usual modes of presentation are:

1. A previously healthy child who is reported to have passed little or no urine for 24 hours or more.
2. The occurrence of oliguria following burns, trauma or operative surgery, or in a child dehydrated from vomiting and diarrhoea.
3. The routine discovery of a raised blood urea level in similar circumstances.

In a previously well child, total anuria suggests obstruction; complete suppression of urine is unusual in both pre-renal and parenchymal failure. Obstruction at or below the bladder neck would be confirmed by the finding of a palpably enlarged bladder, and acute hydronephrosis by a history of loin pain and the discovery of a renal mass on palpation. In the absence of these findings a history of ingesting or inhaling nephrotoxic substances should be sought. Glomerulonephritis is suggested by the absence of antecedents, other than upper respiratory infection in about two thirds of cases. The diagnosis would be supported by the findings of hypertension and raised jugular venous pressure, though both may be absent. The scanty urine would contain protein, erythrocytes and granular casts. If suspected, the diagnosis should be confirmed by percutaneous renal biopsy, which will enable the important distinction to be made between benign and rapidly progressive forms of glomerulonephritis. This procedure carries increased risk in the presence of a rapidly rising blood urea level and should be deferred until the uraemia has been brought under control. The haemolytic-uraemic syndrome occurs mainly in very young children; the renal failure is nearly always preceded by an onset with diarrhoea, but occurs without the severe dehydration which is present when this complication follows gastroenteritis. The diagnosis is confirmed by the finding of a low platelet count, severe haemolytic anaemia and the presence of fragmented erythrocytes and 'burr' cells in blood smears.

The diagnostic problem in the remaining two categories is usually more difficult. The circumstances causing pre-renal failure may lead to ischaemic ATN, and the picture may be further complicated by the existence of a hypercatabolic state. The mere finding of oliguria and a raised blood urea level, singly or together, does not necessarily signify renal failure and is consistent with physiological oliguria. In this state the urine will remain concentrated owing to its high solute content, while increased catabolism will raise both plasma and urine concentrations further. With poor renal perfusion the amount of urea excreted will diminish, although the actual urinary concentration may not necessarily fall below 2 gm/100 ml. In established renal failure, on the other hand, the urinary urea concentration is markedly reduced. Unfortunately there is no clear line of demarcation between pre-renal and renal failure. Measurement of the urinary specific gravity affords a rough guide provided that it is carried out with more than the precision which is possible by floating an unchecked hydrometer in urine contained in a narrow measuring cylinder. Renal function is more closely reflected by the clearance of urea than by the actual urine and plasma concentrations, but since its measurement is impossible in the presence of marked oliguria, the urine/plasma ratio is used as an alternative. The determination of the urine/plasma osmolality ratio is the most reliable test because it takes into account changes in non-urea solutes, in addition to the urea itself. It is simple to perform using a freezing-point osmometer. It is claimed that the production of urine with a low sodium concentration is inconsistent with the presence of ATN, in which high levels are usually found. Finally, the absence of granular casts in the urine, following a careful search, makes renal failure unlikely, but conversely they may be present in the urine of a dehydrated child. The laboratory criteria generally accepted to be of diagnostic significance are summarised in Table 15.4.

Table 15.4 Laboratory criteria generally considered inconsistent with a diagnosis of established renal failure.

1. Urinary S.G.	> 1·022
2. Urinary urea	> 2 gm/100 ml
3. Urine/plasma urea ratio	> 10
4. Urine/plasma osmolality ratio	> 1·1
5. Urinary sodium	> 10 mEq/L
6. Granular casts	absent

Pre-renal failure is a reversible condition which responds to the correction of circulatory insufficiency by the appropriate means, and this is used as the ultimate test to differentiate pre-renal and renal failure. In the absence of such a response the production of an osmotic diuresis by intravenous mannitol infusion will indicate that renal failure, if present, is incipient rather than established.

MANAGEMENT

The decision whether or not to refer the child to a renal unit depends largely upon local factors. While peritoneal dialysis is not beyond the means of a well-staffed district general hospital paediatric unit, there is little doubt that experience in the diagnosis and management of acute renal failure yields superior results. Major burns and cardiac

Acute Renal Failure

surgery units should have such expertise available. Children with primary renal failure who require diagnostic procedures such as renal biopsy should generally be referred to centres specialising in this work.

Obstruction

Before treatment can be ordered, a careful assessment of the diagnosis, as outlined previously, is mandatory. If obstruction is suggested, a plain abdominal radiograph may demonstrate renal enlargement due to hydronephrosis, and possibly calculi. When the bladder is palpably enlarged it should be drained by catheterisation, but the catheter should not initially be left *in situ* because of the risk of infection. Rectal examination may reveal faecal impaction, requiring an enema. Suspicion of an organic obstruction would indicate referral to a urological surgeon.

Pre-renal Failure

The possibility of pre-renal failure will be determined by the circumstances, and the criteria outlined in Table 15.4 should be examined. Catheterisation may be necessary for microscopical and biochemical examination of the urine, as a drowsy child may not void the small quantity of urine present in the bladder. Hypovolaemia should be treated vigorously by the administration of intravenous fluids. In the case of dehydration, normal or hypotonic saline would be used, according to the plasma sodium level, while combinations of blood and plasma are indicated following burns or trauma. This treatment should be continued until the circulatory volume and blood pressure have been restored to normal. The prompt onset of a diuresis will eliminate the diagnosis of renal failure. If doubt remains, renal function should be challenged with more normal or hypotonic saline, with special care to avoid overhydration should no diuresis occur. Danger signs are restlessness, dyspnoea, a raised central venous pressure and basal pulmonary crepitations. Attempts to force a diuresis using intravenous saline in the presence of ATN, are highly dangerous. If there is no response, a therapeutic trial of intravenous mannitol should be conducted, a dose of 0·75 gm/Kg body weight being given as 20 per cent solution over a period of about 5 minutes. If this solution contains crystals at room temperature it should be gently warmed before use. Accurate measurement of the urine flow rate is necessary and urine is usually collected by means of an indwelling catheter, with full aseptic precautions. If the flow rate increases within 3 hours to about 25 ml/M²/hour (or 1 ml/Kg/hour for older children, and nearer 1·5 ml/Kg/hour for infants), fluid administration can safely be continued and further mannitol may be given as 10 per cent solution. If, on the other hand there is no response, this line of treatment should be abandoned after one further attempt; indeed, if the criteria listed in Table 15.4 are indicative of established renal failure, it is doubtful whether even this is justified, for if the child is unable to excrete the mannitol, which is not metabolised, it will cause cellular dehydration and interstitial oedema.

Renal Failure

Water and electrolyte balance
The aim of treatment, once renal failure has become established, is to prevent gross aberrations in the volume and composition of body fluid. The basic fluid requirement is calculated to allow for insensible loss through the skin and lungs, less the amount contributed to body water by tissue catabolism. In children a figure of 250 ml/M²/24 hours is generally accepted as realistic; this is roughly equivalent to 10 ml/Kg/24 hours for older children and 12–15 ml/Kg/24 hours for infants. To this should be added an amount equal to the previous day's urine output plus estimated losses from diarrhoea and vomiting, high fever or excessive sweating. Urine should be collected by means of plastic bags in either sex, or Paul's tubing in the case of boys, if the child is incontinent. Undoubtedly the best way of monitoring progress is by frequent weighing, and a weighing bed is a great convenience. Because of continuing tissue catabolism, a child maintained in ideal fluid balance will lose weight at the rate of approximately 0·5 gm/Kg/24 hours or more when intensely hypercatabolic; attempts to prevent this weight loss will inevitably cause oedema. Fluid given should be electrolyte-free; the dilutional nature of the hyponatraemia is again emphasised.

Nutrition
Adequate calories must be given to minimise protein catabolism, in the form of a flavoured glucose concentrate ('Hycal', Beecham

Acute Renal Failure

Laboratories), each bottle of which supplies 425 Calories in 175 ml of fluid. It may have to be given by nasogastric tube if much nausea occurs. A small quantity of first-class protein minimises the patient's need to break down endogenous protein and reduces the rate of rise of blood urea level. Patients tend to feel better and vomit less than they do on a protein-free diet. The protein should be based on egg and milk and given in a quantity of about 10 gm/M^2/24 hours. Patients who are in an intensely hypercatabolic state, associated with severe burns or septicaemia, need greater amounts of protein and calories to prevent wasting, so that intravenous feeding with 'Aminosol' and 'Intralipid' becomes necessary if vomiting or coma preclude the oral or nasogastric routes.

Acidosis

This can be corrected by the oral or intravenous administration of sodium bicarbonate or lactate, but these buffers have the disadvantage of increasing the sodium content of the body fluids. Severe acidosis is best treated by dialysis.

Hyperkalaemia

This is improved by correction of acidosis and the provision of protein-sparing calories, but the situation may be aggravated by tissue breakdown from burns or large collections of pus. Cardiac arrhythmias are heralded by characteristic electrocardiographic changes as outlined in Chapter 4, so that regular E.C.G. recordings should be made if the plasma potassium level approaches 7 mEq/L. An ion-exchange resin (calcium Resonium) may be given orally or rectally, but tends to aggravate gastrointestinal disturbances. If hyperkalaemia cannot be contained, dialysis is indicated. A rapidly rising plasma potassium level, with E.C.G. changes, may call for emergency intravenous treatment with either soluble insulin and 50 per cent dextrose, sodium bicarbonate or calcium gluconate.

Anaemia

A haemoglobin level of 10 gm/100 ml or more requires no treatment, but severe anaemia which carries the risk of cardiac failure should be corrected by means of small blood transfusions. There is a tendency for the haemoglobin level to stabilise around 10 gm/100 ml and attempts to raise it to much higher levels may be met by haemolysis, with consequent exacerbation of nitrogen and potassium retention. Because of the risk of overloading the circulation, packed cells should generally be used. If there is a bleeding tendency fresh blood may be of temporary benefit, but dialysis is the best means of reversing it.

Infection

Uraemic children are prone to infection, which in turn increases tissue catabolism, and the appropriate antibiotic therapy should be applied with vigour. Certain antibiotics which are normally excreted by the kidney must be given in reduced dosage.

Hypertension

This is often a feature of severe acute glomerulonephritis, but in other forms of renal failure is largely related to sodium and water retention. The best anti-hypertensive drug in renal failure is bethanidine, because of its short action. It should be started in a dose of 5–10 mg according to size, and increased until the blood pressure is controlled. Hypertension may to some extent be a compensatory mechanism for the reduced GFR, and it is advisable not to attempt to reduce the diastolic pressure below 90 mm Hg.

Drugs

It must be remembered that certain drugs which are normally excreted unaltered by the kidneys may reach dangerous blood concentrations if given in conventional dosage. These include sulphonamides, streptomycin, gentamycin, kanamycin, digoxin and phenobarbitone. Penicillin may be given in normal dosage, while short-acting barbiturates, nitrazepam, chloral hydrate and dichloralphenazone are suitable drugs for sedation. Chlorpromazine and promethazine may be given in normal dose, but not repeatedly, owing to cumulative effects. Cyclizine hydrochloride is a safe and effective anti-emetic for oral or intramuscular administration.

DIALYSIS

Indications

Recommended criteria for dialysis are outlined in Table 15.5, but they should not be applied inflexibly. Frequent review of the child's

Acute Renal Failure

general condition is necessary, while the rate of deterioration of biochemical changes is more important than the actual figures. Dialysis should generally be started much earlier in children with extensive burns, for example, than with acute glomerulonephritis, in which the daily blood urea increments may be quite small with conservative management.

Table 15.5 Indications for dialysis.

1. Blood urea	> 400 mg/100 ml
2. Plasma bicarbonate	< 15 mEq/L
3. Plasma potassium	> 8 mEq/L
4. E.C.G. changes of hyperkalaemia	
5. Severely hypercatabolic state	
6. Uncontrollable hypertension	
7. Overhydration	
8. Persistent bleeding tendency	
9. Clinical deterioration, with twitching or convulsions	

Choice of Method

This lies between peritoneal dialysis and haemodialysis. Haemodialysis requires costly apparatus and 24-hour medical and nursing supervision; its efficiency carries with it a greater risk of cerebral disequilibrium, by removing urea from the blood so quickly that an osmotic gradient is set up between cells and extracellular fluid, leading to intracellular oedema. On the other hand it is more effective in severely hypercatabolic patients, and is the method of choice when septicaemia is due to peritonitis. Because of the infrequent need for haemodialysis in children with acute renal failure, few paediatric centres possess the facilities and the method will not be discussed further. For most purposes peritoneal dialysis is effective; it is also cheaper and requires rather less supervision. Where the risk of bleeding is great, either from uraemia or from the use of heparin therapy in treating the haemolytic-uraemic syndrome, it is the method of choice.

Technique of Peritoneal Dialysis

The procedure should be explained to the older child, and a nervous child should be suitably sedated. The bladder must be empty. Meticulous asepsis is necessary. After assembling the delivery set and preparing the skin, a midline site roughly midway between the umbilicus and symphysis pubis is infiltrated with 1 per cent lignocaine. A stab incision is made in the skin through which a 'Trocath' (McGaw Laboratories, Inc.) is introduced, the procedure being facilitated if the abdominal muscles are tensed. After piercing the parietal peritoneum, the stilette is removed and the catheter is pushed gently into the pelvis, as far as it will go. If the pelvis is too shallow, in small infants, the catheter is instead threaded up towards either flank. If difficulty is experienced in inserting the catheter, a quantity of prewarmed dialysing fluid should be run into the peritoneum through an intramuscular needle and a further attempt made. After testing the patency of the catheter by running in a little dialysing fluid, it is secured to the abdominal wall by strips of adhesive plaster over a sterile dressing. If the stab incision is small, sutures will not be needed. The protruding portion of the catheter is trimmed to about 5 cm with sterile scissors before the right-angle connecting tube supplied with it is fitted.

The dialysis system is shown in Fig. 15.1. Only teenagers are likely to accommodate the 2 litres of fluid usually given to adults and, in the case of younger children, one of the pair of supply tubes feeding the drip chamber is clamped and not used. After flushing the system with dialysing fluid, it is connected to the catheter and the fluid is run in with the appropriate clamps wide open. There is no formula for the amount of fluid administered; small infants may only accommodate 150–200 ml, while 10–12 years old children will generally take 1 litre. The right amount is judged in individual patients by the abdominal tension and complaints of marked discomfort. Care must be taken to avoid embarrassing diaphragmatic movement in small infants. Where less than 1 litre will be given in each cycle, bottles of fluid should be used rather than bags since they are calibrated. The first delivery of fluid should be drained immediately, to ensure that the system is working properly. In subsequent cycles the fluid is allowed to remain in the peritoneal cavity for 30 minutes before being drained.

Dialysis fluid preparations all contain physiological amounts of sodium, chloride, calcium and magnesium, together with 45 mEq/L of lactate and are supplied with either 1·36–1·5 per cent or 6·36–7·0 per cent dextrose. The former only produces a small negative fluid balance; the latter is used when patients are overhydrated or suffering from pulmonary oedema and it is desirable to extract larger amounts

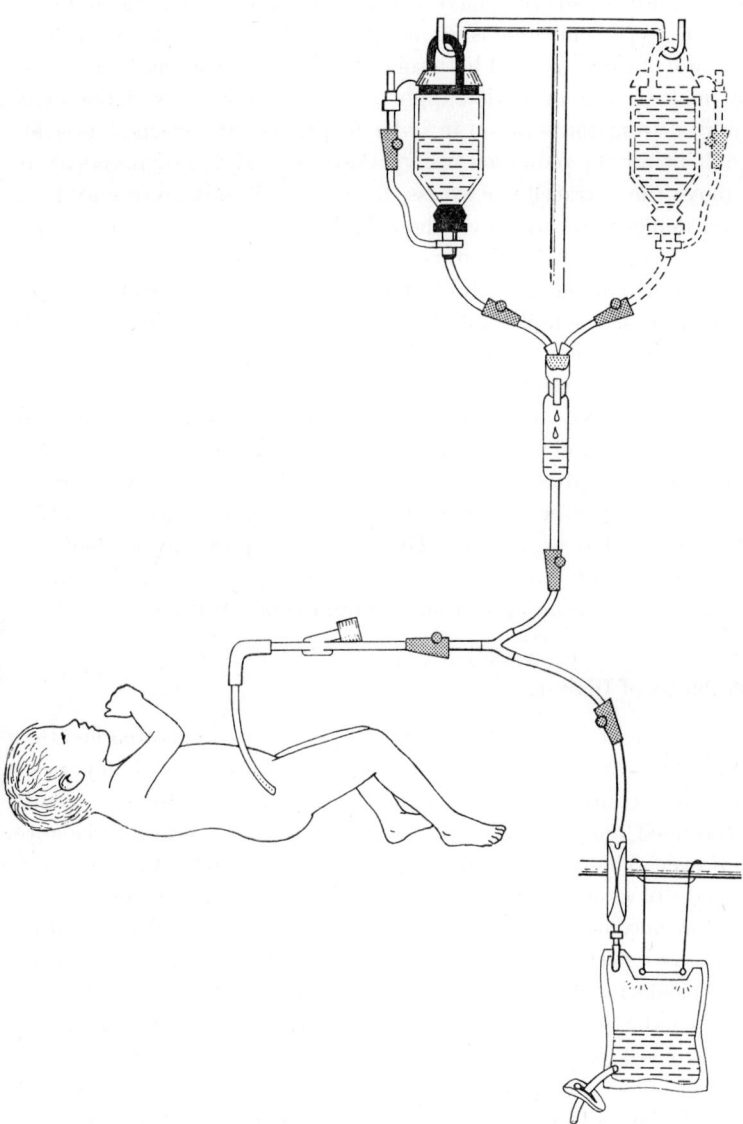

Fig. 15.1 Diagram of Peritoneal Dialysis.

of extracellular fluid from the body. Since most children with acute renal failure are likely to have a surplus of fluid by the time dialysis is started, hypertonic fluid is commonly used for the first 1–2 cycles or a mixture of equal parts of both solutions, which can easily be achieved by making use of both supply tubes. Potassium is deliberately omitted from the solution in order to produce the steepest possible gradient for the reduction of hyperkalaemia. It is only necessary to remove the extracellular excess, for the total body store may have been depleted owing to catabolism. This may be achieved in 4–6 hours, after which 4 mEq of potassium (as chloride) should be added to each litre of dialysing fluid. 500 units of heparin are added to each litre of fluid. A sample of dialysate is cultured bacteriologically daily and any infection treated with the appropriate antibiotic, intraperitoneally or systemically.

Dialysis is used continuously until the plasma electrolytes are more or less normal and the blood urea level is below 100 mg/100 ml, after which daytime dialysis, with a rest at night, is generally sufficient. Treatment, whether conservative or dialytic, is continued until a diuresis becomes established. This may develop rapidly and polyuria may occur, with substantial urinary sodium wastage, and a careful check on hydration and plasma sodium concentration is essential.

Problems of Dialysis

During the first 1–3 cycles the volume of dialysate is often less than that of the dialysing fluid administered, even when the 6·36 per cent dextrose solution is used, so that a positive fluid balance results. Continued dialysis will eventually lead to a net negative balance, however. The dialysate may also be visibly blood stained initially, especially when the stronger solution is used. Diminution or cessation of flow may be due to a number of factors, including blockage of the catheter's perforations by fibrin or blood clot, or by the omentum, and loculation of fluid. The defect can usually be rectified by changing the child's posture, repositioning the catheter, syringing it with heparinised saline, or replacing it with a fresh one. Pain may occur from loculation of fluid or over-distension of the abdomen. Intestinal perforation is fortunately a rare complication. Estimates of the protein content of peritoneal dialysate reveal that children may lose 10–30 gm per day, thus adding to the malnutrition associated with uraemia. While a child is on dialysis therapy, the opportunity should be taken to give a high calorie intake and to promote a positive nitrogen balance by feeding first class protein. Despite these occasional problems, peritoneal dialysis has considerably improved the outlook for children with acute renal failure.

FURTHER READING

BERLYNE, G. M., BAZZARD, F. J., BOOTH, E. M., JANABI, K. & SHAW, A. B. (1967) The dietary treatment of acute renal failure. *Quart. J. Med.*, **36**, 59.

CAMERON, J. S. & MILLER-JONES, C. M. H. (1967) Renal function and renal failure in badly burned children. *Brit. J. Surg.*, **54**, 132.

GALLAGHER, L. & POLAK, A. (1967) The Management of acute renal failure. *Hosp. Med.* (January 1967), p. 287.

MONCRIEFF, M. W., & GLASGOW, E. F., (1970) Haemolytic-uraemic syndrome treated with heparin. *Brit. Med. J.*, **3**, 188.

OGG, C. S., & CAMERON, J. S. (1969) Cardiovascular surgery and the kidney. *Guy's Hosp. Rep.*, **118**, 85.

SHARPSTONE, P. (1970) Acute renal failure. *Brit. Med. J.*, **3**, 158.

WHITE, R. H. R. (1970) Glomerulonephritis in children. *Brit. J. Hosp. Med.*, Vol. 3, p. 746.

CHAPTER

16

Special Problems of Neonates

The normal neonate is at risk from his environment for several reasons, the chief of which are:
1. The temperature-regulating mechanism is unstable so that he can easily either overheat or become hypothermic.
2. The airway is critically small so that obstruction is readily produced by accumulation of bronchial secretions.
3. Defence mechanisms against microbial invasion are not yet efficient so that a severe infection is liable to be followed by septicaemia. Moreover, broad spectrum antibiotic therapy may leave the path open to systemic invasion by monilia.
4. While the infant's kidney can handle water satisfactorily, there is some evidence to suggest that sodium excretion continues despite body sodium depletion.
5. The central nervous system is unstable, and insults to it (e.g. hyperpyrexia, water intoxication, hypoxia) are not infrequently accompanied by convulsions.
6. Body metabolic processes are frequently not efficient during the first few days of life leading to biochemical disturbances with possible secondary effects (e.g. occurrence of jaundice, hypoglycaemia, hypocalcaemia).
7. Incompatibilities of blood group may be present between the mother and her infant.

While the above features may affect the progress of the normal infant after birth, their effects are magnified in the case of infants of low birth weight (less than 2·5 Kg), who may be either premature

Special Problems of Neonates

(judged by gestational date) or dysmature (expected gestational date but 'small for date').

Neonatal morbidity and mortality are dominated by respiratory disorders, and an understanding of the normal changes occurring at birth is important. During intrauterine life the lungs have approximately the same volume as they do after aeration, but the airways are filled with fluid. For such a lung to be capable of normal ventilation it is essential that the alveolar cells are able to secrete surfactant at the alveolar–air interface, this having the property of changing surface tension in relation to surface area so that very low surface tensions can be achieved at reduced areas. This action of surfactant prevents closure of the air spaces at the end of the expiration. The appearance of surfactant corresponds to a body weight of 1·2 Kg which is close to the border-line of viability. Insufficient, or inadequately-acting surfactant leads to the difficulties of pulmonary ventilation found in the respiratory distress syndrome described in Chapter 12.

The aeration of the lungs after birth normally depends on the infant taking his first breath, due to forceful contraction of the respiratory muscles, mainly the diaphragm. The fluid present in the lungs prior to birth is partly evacuated by the squeezing of the infant's thorax during delivery, partly lost with expired air after respiration has been established and partly transported from the alveoli via the blood and/or lymphatics.

After birth the infant may fail to breathe, or may take a few breaths and then begin to show inadequacy of ventilation. If there is no rapid response to pharyngeal suction (which should be performed in an aseptic manner) and a slap on the feet, endotracheal intubation and inflation of the lungs with oxygen should be undertaken without delay because of the risk of cerebral damage from hypoxia. As already stressed in Chapter 12 analeptic drugs should not be employed.

If an infant is exhibiting some respiratory difficulty but is not in extremis an APGAR score should be assessed (see Table 16.1). Repeated scores give some measurable indication of progression or otherwise of respiratory distress, but are to be used in conjunction with other evidence, such as determination of acid/base balance, measurement of blood gases, an assessment of the state of the central nervous system (e.g. possibility of intracranial haemorrhage or effect of drugs given to the mother), condition of the cardiovascular system, temperature and presence of cyanosis.

Table 16.1 APGAR scoring for respiratory distress.

	Sign	Score 0	Score 1	Score 2
A	Appearance	Blue or pale	Baby pink, limbs blue	All pink
P	Pulse	Absent	Below 100	Over 100
G	Grimace (reflex response to stimulation of sole of foot)	No response	Grimace	Cry
A	Activity: muscle tone	Limp	Some flexion of limbs	Active movements
R	Respiration	Absent	Slow; irregular	Good strong cry

Assisted respiration in the neonate by means of a facemask and rebreathing bag has to be undertaken with considerable caution because of the danger of distension of the stomach with consequent splinting of the diaphragm and increased difficulty of ventilation. The administration of oxygen via a rubber funnel is only of historical interest.

The care of the respiratory tract in general terms has been discussed in Chapters 9 and 12. However, it must be stressed that the airway in the neonate is already critically small. It will be recalled that gas flow varies as the fourth power of the radius; thus the addition of 0·5 mm of exudate to a trachea of radius 2·0 mm (reducing the radius of the lumen to 1·5 mm) would reduce gas flow three times unless there were an increase of respiratory work. Since thickening of tracheo-bronchial secretions must be prevented by humidification of inspired gas it is important to employ an efficient humidifier. Care must be taken if ultrasonic nebulisers are employed because of the risk of water overload of the baby and daily weighing is important. It is sometimes useful to employ 'local humidification', the inspired gas being led into a small plastic box situated around the infant's head, a crescent being cut out of the box to allow passage of the neck. A disadvantage of this apparatus is the fact that the dense mist makes it difficult to inspect the infant's face.

INCUBATORS AND THE MAINTENANCE OF A STABLE ENVIRONMENT

Undue handling of a neonate is to be avoided, but it is important that he may be observed fully at all times. For this reason it is often desirable for him to be nursed, uncovered, in an incubator which acts as his own cubicle, but this will only be necessary until the acute stage of the illness is over. With regard to observation adequate room lighting must be available at all times; the infants can sleep quite satisfactorily despite twenty-four hour illumination.

One advantage of an incubator, apart from ease of observation, is the maintenance of an even ambient temperature and, indeed, some types of incubator employ a servo mechanism from a thermocouple monitoring the infant's skin or core temperature, so enabling automatic adjustment of the incubator temperature to deal with an abnormal fall or elevation of body temperature. All incubators employ safety cut-out mechanisms to prevent overheating. It is very important to avoid chilling of the infant, particularly if debilitated, dehydrated or premature, as this may be followed by the onset of sclerema, with diffuse hardening of the subcutaneous tissues beginning in the lower limbs and progressing to involve the whole body; most cases have a fatal termination and there is no specific therapy although steroids are said to cause improvement in some patients. It is well known of course that overheating any patient leads to increased oxygen consumption, but it may not be realised that chilling an infant also increases oxygen consumption due to non-shivering heat production as a result of oxidation of brown fat, a process facilitated by increased blood supply to the fat caused by noradrenaline. The infant's oxygen requirements are therefore ciitical with regard to ambient temperature.

Another advantage of an incubator is the ability to circulate air, or oxygen-enriched air, throughout the canopy, but care must be taken in the case of premature babies of low birth weight (under 1·5 Kg) and of gestational age of six to seven months, not to exceed an oxygen concentration of 40 per cent, otherwise permanent blindness may result from retrolental fibroplasia and corneal overgrowth. It is important not to rely on the makers' recommended admixture of oxygen but to check the oxygen concentration with an oximeter. Of course, if the infant's P_aO_2 is low a higher inspired oxygen must be employed, and it is likely that retinal disorders will not follow provided the $P_{a}O_2$ is within normal limits.

Generalised humidity can be provided within the incubator, assisted if necessary by the nebulisation of water. Although this has the advantage of diminishing the viscosity of tracheobronchial secretions, and also reducing insensible water loss, there is a distinct disadvantage in that an environment is provided favourable to the growth of Ps. pyocyanea.

Another disadvantage of incubators is the fact that the infant is contaminating his own environment by the passage of excreta and it is essential to employ frequent changes of incubator (for example every 48 hours) to allow time for cleaning and sterilisation. Contamination of the inside of the incubator can also occur by the insertion of the gowned arms of medical and nursing staff through the port holes. Regular bacteriological examination of such material as pharyngeal or endotracheal suction catheters, umbilical swabs etc. is important, but it is equally important *not* to treat bacteriological reports but to treat the patient. Obviously if a heavy growth of a particular pathogen is obtained from any source it should be treated. Less obvious is the need to resist the temptation to treat the culture of occasional colonies of a pathogen. To do so, particularly with broad spectrum antibiotics, invites the replacement of pyogenic organisms with Ps. pyocyanea, and if this too is eradicated, the path is left open for invasion by fungi, particularly candida albicans, which can assume septicaemic proportions. It is of course important to appreciate that the neonate is at risk from a variety of infections which may spread to involve the lungs, meninges, bones, intestinal or renal tracts. Before there is any definite evidence of localisation of infection the infant may have ceased to feed well, he may be restless or unduly quiet, he may have a tachycardia (less commonly a fever), or an increased respiratory rate. Such warnings must not be neglected and may be the indication for such investigations as blood culture, the examination of the urine and perhaps lumbar puncture.

A further disadvantage of incubators lies in the difficulty of access to the infant for such purposes as the passage of an endotracheal tube, the setting up of an intravenous infusion, or even the positioning of the infant for a satisfactory portable radiological examination. If an incubator is employed it is important that additional holes should be cut in the canopy (covered by plastic 'pear drops' when not being

Special Problems of Neonates

used), suitably sited, to allow the entry of ventilator tubing, and the exit of drainage tubes, monitoring cables and cannulae. Drainage tube holes must be made sufficiently low down to allow dependent drainage. In many instances if an infant requires ventilatory support it is preferable to nurse him in a bassinette with overhead infra-red lamps to avoid loss of body heat.

GENERAL MANAGEMENT

In addition to the usual patient recordings of temperature, pulse and respiratory rate it is frequently important to have warning devices as a safeguard against cardiorespiratory arrest. Infants of low birth weight are prone to episodes of apnoea, and respiratory effort is resumed either spontaneously or after cutaneous stimulation. Prolonged apnoea will result in bradycardia after an initial short period of tachycardia. Apnoea monitors rely either on changes in a thermistor in an air inflated mattress, or on changes in electrical impedance across the chest with inflation of the lungs. No apnoea monitor is entirely satisfactory, the main problem being the frequency of false alarms, and it is preferable to monitor cardiac action by a cardioscope with an audible 'bleep' in addition to respiration. *Such warning devices are an assistance to the nurse and do not replace adequate observation of the patient.* In order to avoid the inconvenience of separate limb electrodes for the cardioscope a disposable 'three-in-one' electrode* may be applied to the front of the chest.

Cannulae inserted into veins or arteries require careful management to avoid displacement, kinking or occlusion by blood clot. Such cannulae are of necessity small, and clotting within the lumen is preferably prevented by periodic injection of a small quantity of heparinized saline. It is usually not practical to have a continuous slow injection of heparinized saline, as the very slow flow is insufficient to prevent clotting.

Drainage tubes must be dependent to allow proper evacuation of exudate etc. In this respect it is important to appreciate that an intercostal tube, attached by a fairly long piece of tubing to an underwater seal drain, results in a situation of paradoxical breathing, and the greater the 'swing' of water level in the tube, the greater is the

* Manufactured by Dracard Limited, Maidstone, Kent.

amount of paradox. It is therefore essential to have suction attached to the drainage bottle to achieve a vacuum of about 10 mm Hg.

Not infrequently after major surgery, or as a complication of infection, there is a period of impaired gastro-intestinal function and ileus. Most infants will continue to make sucking movements (particularly if some foreign object is passing through the mouth such as an endotracheal tube) and will swallow air and saliva. This can result in marked gastric or gastro-intestinal distension, which can seriously embarass diaphragmatic movements and impair pulmonary ventilation. It is important to prevent this complication by passage of a nasogastric tube, sufficiently large to allow easy withdrawal of air, *and this should not be kept occluded by a spigot but should be left open*, intermittent aspiration by syringe being carried out. It is sometimes advisable to keep continuous gentle suction (a vacuum of about 5 mm Hg) on the tube. Any aspirate should be kept and measured, and its nature recorded. It must be stressed that the only *certain* indication that the end of a nasogastric tube is in fact in the stomach is by radiological proof, and such tubes should have a radio-opaque sentinel line down the length (e.g. the Argyle pattern*). The aspiration of material which has an acid reaction to litmus does not prove that the tube is in the stomach as, if the tube is lying in the oesophagus and some gastro-oesophageal regurgitation has taken place, gastric juice is in fact aspirated from the oesophagus.

Temperature recording is very important and to avoid repeated disturbance of the infant may conveniently be done continuously using a thermocouple and electrothermometer. Some difficulty may be experienced as skin and 'core' temperatures are not the same, while recording of intra-oesophageal temperature via an electrode inserted through the nose or mouth tends to provoke excessive oropharyngeal secretions, and an electrode in the rectum may give false readings if it becomes insulated by a layer of faeces.

Collection of the urine is essential in many conditions for an accurate comparison of intake and output, and for measurement of electrolyte and other losses. Urethral catheterisation is to be avoided if possible because of the risk of infection in the urinary tract, and urine may be collected in a plastic bag such as the 'Chironseal'†

* Manufactured by Brunswick Corporation, Worthing, Sussex.

† Manufactured by Down Bros. and Mayer and Phelps Ltd., Mitcham, Surrey.

Special Problems of Neonates

which is fixed to the perineum by adhesive. This does cause some irritation, with a possibility of infection of the skin.

Fluid and Electrolyte Balance, Blood replacement and Nutrition

It is true that the *normal* new born infant requires little in the way of water, electrolyte and Calories in the first day or so of life. However, the presence of infection or congenital anomalies necessitating operation will often be an indication that fluid should be given. In such instances as congenital intestinal obstruction, or hypoglycaemia, it will not be possible to give the required fluid into the gastrointestinal tract and intravenous infusion is necessary, preferably given via a fine needle inserted into a scalp vein and fixed firmly into place. If the umbilical vein is patent a polyethylene catheter can be inserted for administration of fluids but care must be taken to avoid infection and the use of *cold* solutions which may provoke portal vein thrombosis with resulting extrahepatic portal hypertension.

The principles of intravenous fluid therapy have already been discussed in Chapter 4. It must be re-emphasized that parenteral infusions must increase in a linear manner (by sevenths of the total requirement) up to the seventh day of life, with an increased intake if there are abnormal losses. Post-operative infants lose potassium, nitrogen and also magnesium (which closely follows nitrogen) in the urine. The loss of magnesium may have important repercussions if the serum ionized calcium is low, since neonatal tetany resistant to calcium administration may occur. In such circumstances the serum magnesium must be estimated (normal 1·5–2·0 mg/100 ml) and, if low, magnesium sulphate given intramuscularly providing renal function is adequate (dose 0·1–0·4 ml/Kg of 50 per cent solution every 4–6 hours). Phosphates are also lost in the post-operative infant, the amount being related to potassium excretion.

The normal newborn can have a variation of standard bicarbonate between 15 and 27 mEq/L (or base deficit of −12 to base excess of +4 mEq/L). Values outside the normal accepted range for older children therefore do not necessarily indicate abnormalities in acid/base balance but must be assessed in relation to the physical state of the child and other relevant findings. Similarly, the capillary $P\text{co}_2$ of normal infants up to the age of 2 weeks may be within the range of 20–60 mm Hg.

Every endeavour must be made to avoid blood loss during operations on the newborn, and in considering replacement therapy it must be remembered that in the first week of life the haemoglobin in capillary blood is about 20 gm/100 ml while the haematocrit is about 65 c.cm/100 ml, reflecting the 'Mount Everest in utero'. Ideally blood replacement should be controlled by accurate measurement of loss, but in an emergency it is reasonably safe to administer blood to a volume equal to 20 ml of whole blood/Kg of body weight. It is important not to transfuse cold 'bank' blood, but this should be warmed by passage through a coil of tubing immersed in a thermostatically controlled warming tank before it enters the infant's veins. Relatively large volumes of cold blood will cause hypothermia, cardiac irregularities and possibly cardiac arrest. It is also necessary to consider the calcium/potassium imbalance resulting from transfusion, and the production of a metabolic alkalosis from metabolism of citrate.

Nutritional requirements should be supplied by normal feeding whenever possible, using expressed breast milk, or proprietary preparations, if necessary via a nasogastric tube. A parenteral schedule cannot provide a copy of maternal milk because fat can only be given intravenously in a dose of 2 gm/Kg body weight as 'Intralipid'. Premature babies, and babies of low birth weight, require 4–5 gm/Kg of aminoacids with 80–100 Cals/Kg to grow at a rate equivalent to that in utero, and the intake of water should be in the region of 140 ml/100 Cals. Using the infusion solutions described in Chapter 4 by giving carbohydrates to 13 gm/Kg and aminoacids to 2·5 gm/Kg body weight no more than 80 Cals/Kg can be provided, and the amount of nitrogen is insufficient.

THE NEUROLOGICAL STATE OF THE NEONATE

The central nervous system of the normal newborn infant is not yet fully mature. The degree of maturation is retarded by malnutrition, and also by premature birth. Cerebral symptoms may be found in any newborn infant requiring I.T.U. admission, and may be transient in nature. Investigation of such symptoms requires a knowledge of asphyxia (both prenatal and following delivery), and examination of the infant with regard to his general condition, position and move-

Special Problems of Neonates

ments, muscular tone, Moro reflex, ability to suck and to ventilate his lungs adequately.

The aetiological factors of convulsions are numerous, and these may appear as typical grand mal attacks or episodes of intermittent cyanosis with tonic extension of the body. The commonest causes are:

1. Cerebral birth trauma.
2. Hypoxia.
3. Developmental defects of the nervous system.
4. Infection of the brain and/or meninges.
5. Pyrexia (e.g. due to acute otitis media).
6. Metabolic upsets, e.g. hypoglycaemia.
7. Fluid and electrolyte disturbances (e.g. water intoxication hypocalcaemia, hyponatraemia).

Specific cerebral symptoms include convulsions, tremor, rigidity, and restlessness and irritability. The clinical picture may fall into one of the following groups, which are not necessarily clear cut:

(a) *The one-sided syndrome*, with decreased movements on one side, an asymmetrical position and Moro reflex, differing muscle tone on the two sides and a history of difficult delivery.

(b) *The hyperexcitability syndrome*, with hypermobility and hyper-irritability (the 'jittery' baby), increased low frequency tremor, hypertonic muscles with exaggerated reflexes, and an increased Moro reflex. This state is suspicious of asphyxia, and may also be associated with metabolic or electrolyte disturbances.

(c) *The rigidity syndrome*, in which there are defective spontaneous movements, a position of opisthotonus, gross extension hypertonicity with a marked tonic neck reflex, and a pathological flexion Moro reflex. This may occur after asphyxia, or in association with severe jaundice.

(d) *The 'floppy infant' syndrome*, where the infant is apathetic, showing reduced movements and hypotonic muscles, with a poor or absent Moro reflex, and poor sucking movement and crying. The 'frog position' may be adopted, and there may be no relevant history of trauma, asphyxia etc.

Hypoglycaemia with a blood sugar level below 20 mg per cent may be very serious if convulsions occur, as the possibility of permanent severe brain damage is high. It is a particular hazard of the small dysmature infant, and requires the urgent intravenous administration of 50 per cent dextrose (1–2 ml/Kg of body weight) together with a maintenance infusion of 10 per cent dextrose or 20 per cent laevulose at a rate of 5 ml/Kg of body weight/hour. It may be necessary to give steroids such as prednisone 0·5 mg/Kg two or three times daily.

Hypocalcaemia occurring in the newborn may be due to the fact that the parathyroid glands are not very efficient so that the infant has a functional hypoparathyroidism and has difficulty in mobilising calcium from his skeleton. If feeding with cow's milk formulae is introduced, the relatively high phosphate intake may cause disturbances in calcium/phosphorus balance and tetany or convulsions may result. In some infants hypocalcaemic convulsions occur before oral feeding has been commenced. The serum calcium is below 7 mg per cent and the phosphorus is usually above this level. Combined hypocalcaemia and hypoglycaemia is particularly damaging to the brain.

Treatment should be initially by slow intravenous injection of calcium gluconate 30 mg/Kg of body weight (0·3 ml/Kg of 10 per cent solution diluted to 2·5 per cent with water), and this may have to be repeated. Calcium chloride may be added to gastric feeds (50 mg/Kg of body weight, three to four times daily) together with vitamin D, but resistant hypocalcaemia may indicate hypomagnesaemia which requires treatment as already described.

SOME SPECIAL CONDITIONS IN NEONATES

The Respiratory Distress Syndrome

This has already been outlined in Chapter 12.

Congenital Oesophageal Abnormalities

Most of such infants have a blind upper oesophagus with a communication between the trachea and the distal oesophagus (tracheo-oesophageal fistula). Some have only atresia without any communication between the respiratory and alimentary tract, while others have an 'H-shaped' tracheo-oesophageal fistula without oesophageal obstruction. In all patients the object of treatment is to preserve the integrity of the respiratory tract, while reconstruction of the alimentary tract is a secondary consideration. In the commonest variety of abnormality the infant is at risk from inhalation of oro-pharyngeal secretions from the upper oesophagus, while gastro-oesophago-

Special Problems of Neonates

tracheal regurgitation through the fistula will lead to Mendelson's syndrome. Preoperatively, therefore, it is important to protect the infant from both of these risks by nursing him *head down*, with a 10°–15° tilt of the incubator mattress. The risk of contamination of the lungs by gastric juice does not exist in 'pure' oesophageal atresia, but is perhaps a risk in the case of tracheo-oesophageal fistula without atresia. Gastric distension is often marked where a communication exists between the oesophagus and trachea, and is an obvious embarrassment to proper pulmonary ventilation both pre-operatively and at operation.

The main need in treating such infants post-operatively is the necessity to preserve lung function. Gastric distension must be prevented by nasogastric suction to allow adequate diaphragmatic movement, and there should be no hesitation to introduce an orotracheal tube for bronchial lavage, suction and hand ventilation of the lungs if respiratory distress is due to retention of bronchial secretions; this may have to be repeated, and if necessary the tube can be left in the trachea for 24–48 hours. Mendelson's syndrome is managed as described in Chapter 12.

Congenital Diaphragmatic (Pleuro-peritoneal) Hernia

In this condition the lung on one side is compressed and collapsed by intestines, present in the pleural cavity during intrauterine life, which have distended with gas after the infant has swallowed air. The presence of the intestines causes interference with normal growth of the lung on the side of the hernia, and this is thus hypoplastic, while in gross herniae both lungs may be small. Post-operative difficulties with pulmonary function are therefore due to the hypoplastic nature of one or both lungs, and the splinting effect on the diaphragm of the mass of intestines, these being contained now within an abdominal cavity which is too small for them. It is thus most important to limit gastro-intestinal distension by nasogastric suction and to withhold gastric feeds until good bowel function is established, while inadequate ventilation may have to be assisted by mechanical means. The latter must be used with great care because of the danger of rupture of the hypoplastic lung or lungs with consequent tension pneumothorax, a complication which requires urgent recognition and relief by the insertion of intercostal drainage tubes.

Jaundice

Some degree of jaundice occurs in all new born infants ('physiological' jaundice) and reflects the inability of the immature liver to deal with bile pigment resulting from the normal destruction of superfluous red cells. The jaundice usually clears fairly rapidly over a period of several days. However, if jaundice occurs in a baby in the I.T.U. the serum bilirubin should be estimated daily, because levels of indirect bilirubin exceeding 20 mg per cent may cause brain damage (kernicterus) *whatever the cause of the jaundice may be* and are usually an indication for exchange transfusion. Investigation is also necessary to exclude Rhesus or A–B–O incompatibility between the baby and his mother. Other causes of jaundice are prematurity, bacterial infection, hypothyroidism, galactosaemia, hepatitis and atresia of the bile ducts, all of which may complicate the condition for which I.T.U. admission was necessary.

Cardiac Problems

Most infants admitted to an I.T.U. with heart diseases will have had operations to help heart failure by improving oxygenation, or decreasing or abolishing a left-to-right shunt, or decreasing ventricular work by relieving an obstruction of the right or left ventricle.

In the first week or so of life hypoxia due to heart disease is likely to be due to the Fallot variety of defect, or to transposition of the great arteries. Where pulmonary blood flow is reduced, as in the baby with tetralogy of Fallot, an aorto-pulmonary shunt gives the best chance of survival. Palliation of transposition depends on getting adequate mixing of right and left atrial blood by the creation of an atrial septal defect, either at cardiac catheterisation (balloon septostomy) or in the operating theatre (Blalock-Hanlon operation, or open atrial septostomy). In both of these varieties of cyanotic heart disease there is usually a severe metabolic acidosis requiring correction, and care must be taken to assess kidney function and to prevent dehydration.

Left-to-right shunts are treated where possible by curative procedures, for example, ligation of a persistent ductus arteriosus. If abolition of the shunt is not possible (because, for example, of the difficulty of open heart procedures on a tiny infant) pulmonary blood flow is reduced by pulmonary artery banding. Following this, pulmonary compliance *may* improve fairly rapidly, but persisting ventilatory difficulties not infrequently require a period of artificial ventilation of the lungs.

'Pure' right ventricular obstruction due to valvular stenosis is sometimes seen in infancy and usually causes some right-to-left shunting through a 'forced' foramen ovale, with arterial hypoxaemia and a metabolic acidosis sufficiently severe to cause cardiac arrest. Operative relief of the obstruction leads to a dramatic improvement of cardiac output and a prolonged post-operative admission to the I.T.U. is not usually necessary. However, left ventricular obstructions (usually coarctation of the aorta, with an accompanying left-to-right shunt through a persistent ductus or ventricular septal defect) require surgery when the infant is in cardiac failure, resistant to medical treatment, with hepatomegaly, a raised central venous pressure, pulmonary congestion and possibly pulmonary oedema. The pulmonary compliance is always reduced and remains so for a time after operation so that mechanical ventilation of the lungs is frequently necessary.

CHAPTER 17

Convulsive States and the Unconscious Patient

CARE OF THE UNCONSCIOUS PATIENT

In the context of intensive therapy, this refers to a patient kept still or paralysed by drugs and ventilated for treatment of specific conditions, as well as to those unconscious from other causes. These patients are all unable to feed themselves, are usually incontinent and are unable to move voluntarily in response to painful stimuli. Care must therefore encompass the whole patient.

The Airway

An unconscious patient usually has a diminished or absent cough reflex, and the lungs are in danger from inhalation of saliva or vomitus. If the patient is supine, the tongue will fall back, occluding the pharynx and causing airway obstruction. In an emergency, the first treatment of a patient unconscious from any cause is to clear the mouth of any material, preferably by suction, and to turn the patient into a semi-prone position, so that the lower jaw and tongue fall forward, relieving airway obstruction. If turning is inconvenient, the jaw should be held forward, and the head extended at the atlanto-occipital joint, a Guedel airway being inserted if needed. If the patient is not breathing, steps must be taken to ventilate the lungs, by face mask or endotracheal tube. If inhalation of stomach contents is suspected, bronchial lavage with saline should be carried out without delay.

Long term unconsciousness, as may result from head injury, will result in inadequate coughing and clearing of secretions, and an endotracheal tube or tracheostomy may be needed to prevent pulmonary collapse and infection. Humidification of such an artificial airway is, of course, essential, and suction must be performed with care, to minimise the introduction of infection. Frequent turning of the patient, and physiotherapy, will be needed to prevent segmental collapse of the lung due to secretions. It is recommended that at some time the patient should be turned almost prone to assist drainage of the posterior parts of the lungs. Inadequate respiration must be treated with artificial ventilation, as has been described, provided there is some prospect of recovery.

Cerebral oedema may be lessened by hyperventilation of the lungs, provided the mean intrathoracic pressure is kept low, by the employment of a negative pressure during expiration. This is only feasible if the lungs are normal. Hypocapnia is also thought by some to be beneficial in the presence of brain damage, as there is experimental evidence to suggest a paradoxical increase of blood supply to damaged areas of brain in the presence of a respiratory alkalosis.

Hydration and Nutrition

Adequate hydration is essential and should be maintained by intragastric tube or intravenous infusion, depending on bowel function. The intragastric route is to be preferred if possible. Proper hydration also assists in the care of the airway, as bronchial secretions are kept moist. In the presence of dehydration, intravenous fluids should be used initially to accomplish rehydration.

In the treatment of cerebral oedema, or overdosage of some drugs, diuretics may be required. Intravenous mannitol is preferred, given as a 20 per cent solution in a dosage of 1 gm/Kg over the course of half an hour. This drug is an osmotic diuretic, and induces a transient increase in circulating blood volume. It is thought to improve renal blood flow slightly, so may be of use in impending renal failure. If cardiac failure is present, frusemide is the diuretic of choice.

In considering the total daily intake of fluid, renal function and the insensible fluid loss must be taken into account, and the latter may be less than is expected if an artificial airway is being fully humidified.

There may also be losses from gastric aspirate, and any electrolyte imbalance must be corrected.

The urine must be collected, partly as a record of fluid output, and partly to keep the bed dry. This can be difficult, especially in babies. If possible it is best to avoid urethral catheterisation, due to the hazard of introducing infection. A receptacle must be fixed to the penis in the male, and the perineum in the female. This is usually a plastic bag with a sticky area in infants and older girls. In older boys a rubber sheath may be fixed to the penis by adhesive strapping. With any of these methods there is a tendency to develop soreness and ulceration of the skin.

Maintenance of nutrition is very important, as nitrogen is lost and muscle wasting occurs, in any person lying in bed. As soon as possible, a high Calorie intake must be provided. If the bowel is functioning, the gastric route is much to be preferred. Usually a nasogastric tube is used in the first instance, but a feeding gastrostomy or jejunostomy may be preferred in the long term. Careful attention must, of course, be paid to bowel function, and the prevention of constipation, or the fluid and electrolyte losses associated with diarrhoea, is important. In the early stages of the illness, acute gastric dilatation may occur, and, if undetected, may cause death from regurgitation and inhalation. If a nasogastric tube is used, it should be aspirated before feeds, to ensure that fluid is being absorbed, and that the tube is still in the stomach. In acute illness, especially if there is abdominal distension, the tube should drain continuously, the fluid losses being measured and replaced intravenously. If the bowel is not functioning, Calories must be provided intravenously, but this has some disadvantages, as described in Chapter 4.

The Skin

The health of the skin depends on its having adequate tissue oxygenation, and in an unconscious patient there is a danger of diminished blood supply to the areas of skin in contact with the bed, especially those bearing weight. This becomes a worse problem in patients with low cardiac output and hypoxaemia. After a time, weight-bearing areas normally become painful, and the conscious person would change his position. Therefore the body position of an unconscious patient must be changed routinely every two hours, in regular rotation, so that no area of skin is unduly compressed. The importance of this cannot be over-stressed, as ulceration of the skin over pressure areas is very hard to treat, and should be prevented. Attention to general nutrition is also important in the preservation of the integrity of the skin.

The 'pressure areas', that is, weight bearing areas where bone is close to the skin, such as the sacrum, spine, elbows and heels, should be inspected carefully for redness, stasis being eliminated and the blood supply encouraged by massage. It is very important that the skin be kept clean and dry, and sheets be kept as wrinkle-free as possible. Some assistance can be gained from the use of 'ripple' mattresses, which constantly change the area of bed in contact with skin, or by using a sheepskin, which is soft, and helps to keep the skin dry.

Equally important is the prevention of pressure being applied to points where nerves are vulnerable, such as the ulnar nerve at the elbow and the lateral popliteal nerve at the upper end of the fibula.

The cornea must be prevented from drying, by keeping the eyes closed, or by instilling oily drops, otherwise painful corneal ulceration will occur with the danger of infection.

Joints which are not moved will become stiff, hands tend to become oedematous, and foot drop may occur if the feet are left unsupported and subjected to the weight of bed clothes. Physiotherapy therefore plays an essential part in preventing deformity by putting joints through their range of movement daily, exercising the hands, and stimulating inactive muscles to help prevent wasting. Foot splints may be necessary.

THE CAUSES OF UNCONSCIOUSNESS

The unconscious state may be due to a variety of causes some of which are:

Central Nervous System
- (i) idiopathic   e.g. epilepsy
- (ii) congenital   e.g. hydrocephalus
- (iii) traumatic   e.g. head injury, or hypoxia following cardiac arrest or drowning
- (iv) thermal   e.g. febrile convulsions in infants, or hyperpyrexia

(v) infective   e.g. meningitis, encephalitis
(vi) vascular   e.g. arterial or venous thrombosis or haemorrhage
(vii) neoplastic   e.g. raised intracranial tension from tumours

Metabolic
   (i) diabetic ketoacidosis
   (ii) hypoglycaemia
   (iii) hypercarbia
   (iv) hyponatraemia
   (v) hypocalcaemia
   (vi) liver failure
   (vii) renal failure

Hormonal
   (i) hypothyroidism
   (ii) hypopituitarism
   (iii) adrenal failure

Drug overdosage
   (i) barbiturates and other hypnotics
   (ii) aspirin
   (iii) tranquillisers etc.

Psychosis

In differentiating the many causes of coma, a history of its onset is very important, as is a thorough physical examination and relevant investigations which include examination of the blood for serum electrolytes, urea, blood gas tensions, sugar, and drugs; lumbar puncture in the absence of papilloedema; measurement of the 'core' body temperature (oesophageal or rectal); radiographic examination as indicated, electroencephalography. Some conditions will be discussed in more detail.

Convulsive States in General

Convulsions may originate from a variety of sources—from a focus of irritation within the brain, either 'idiopathic' or following trauma, hypoxia, or neoplasm; from high temperatures in children, usually due to infection of the ears or throat, but sometimes as an abnormal reaction to drugs; from electrolyte disturbances, usually a low serum sodium or ionised calcium, or the combination of the latter with hypoglycaemia in neonates; from irritation of the spinal cord as in tetanus; or associated with drug overdosage (notably aspirin in children, tranquillisers or atropine).

The originating cause must be sought and treated, but all these patients share the danger of hypoxia. Convulsing muscles consume large amounts of oxygen and this is increased if there is fever. Generalised convulsions interfere with respiration, so uptake of oxygen is impaired. The body carries no effective stores of oxygen, and there is increased extraction of oxygen from the blood, with the production of a metabolic acidosis from anaerobic metabolism. This will not occur rapidly unless ventilation is grossly impaired, but the danger lies in the insidious onset of hypoxia, which may be overlooked, with the possibility of cerebral damage.

Conventional treatment of status epilepticus includes the use of such cerebral depressant drugs as phenobarbitone, phenytoin, paraldehyde, thiopentone, and normal doses of such drugs should be tried. However, these drugs also depress the respiratory centre, and if a reasonable dose fails to control the convulsions, then measures should be taken to improve oxygenation, rather than to increase the dose of respiratory depressant drug. Diazepam has been found useful in controlling fits in some cases, and does not depress respiration, except in large doses.

Oxygenation may be ensured by the use of muscle relaxants, endotracheal intubation and artificial ventilation of the lungs until the fits stop. Cerebral depressant drugs may be continued, although it is doubtful if any real benefit is gained. The problem is, of course, then to discover when the convulsions actually stop, while valuable neurological signs may be lost. However, the benefits of adequate oxygenation outweigh these disadvantages. If hypoxia is allowed to develop, cerebral irritation is increased and the fits made worse. Repeat doses of muscle relaxant are not normally given until signs of movement are present, and convulsive movements can usually be distinguished. If neurological examination is essential, the effects of the relaxant may be allowed to wear off for a time.

Electrolyte Disturbances

Convulsions due to such disturbances are amenable to treatment if the cause is recognised. Hyponatraemia (excluding that due to chronic cardiac failure) leads to cerebral oedema and may cause convulsions if the serum sodium falls below 120 mEq/L. It is seen occasionally post-operatively in neonates, the cause being unknown, but perhaps the neonatal kidney fails to conserve sodium. It may also occur after cardio-pulmonary bypass. The treatment is administration of hypertonic saline intravenously which will cause a diuresis, provided renal function is normal.

The level of *ionised* serum calcium is important from the point of view of nerve irritability. Total calcium may fall, due to deficient intake, deficient absorption from the bowel, parathyroid deficiency, or chronic nephritis. Ionised serum calcium will fall in the presence of an alkalosis, either metabolic or respiratory. Hypocalcaemia causes convulsions and laryngeal stridor in children, but not usually in adults. Carpopedal spasm may be seen in all age groups. Treatment is of the original cause, but the immediate situation can be relieved by giving a slow intravenous injection of 10 per cent calcium gluconate. Nerve irritability also depends on the serum magnesium level, which should be measured if the hypocalcaemia is refractory to treatment, especially in infants.

Tetanus

The causative organism is the anaerobic bacillus, Clostridium tetani, which infects a wound contaminated by soil, usually a puncture wound or compound fracture, in which oxygenation is poor. Often the original wound is very small and may pass unnoticed. An open wound, or conversion of a closed to an open one, will kill the bacillus. Neonatal tetanus occasionally occurs, from infection of the umbilical cord. The incubation period varies from a few days to several weeks, and in general it may be said that the disease is more severe after a short incubation period. The bacilli produce a toxin which travels along the peri-neural lymphatics, to reach the spinal cord, where it causes irritability of the anterior horn cells. This leads to intermittent muscle spasm, which may affect only the involved limb, or the whole body, in which case severe opisthotonus occurs, the spasm sometimes being severe enough to cause fractures.

The disease may be divided into mild, moderate, or severe forms. In its mild form there may be only localised spasm of the infected

Convulsive States and the Unconscious Patient

limb, or infrequent, more generalised spasms. Management will require sedation and bed rest.

Moderate tetanus involves generalised muscular spasms, five or six a day, which do not cause much hypoxia, and can be treated by sedation and the use of the spinal muscle relaxant, mephanesin.

Severe tetanus usually occurs after a short incubation period, and the muscle spasms are severe enough to require treatment by muscle paralysis, tracheostomy and artificial ventilation with an air-oxygen mixture. Such treatment may be required for several weeks and care of the airway and lungs must be meticulous. Penicillin is given, and the wound is opened. The use of anti-tetanic serum is controversial because it may lead to a severe anaphylactic reaction. Probably it is better omitted, because the patient will soon develop his own antibodies.

The mortality of severe tetanus even treated by this method has been high, and investigation has shown that there is often associated overactivity of the sympathetic nervous system. Relatively small stimuli, such as endotracheal suction, can cause extreme rises in blood pressure and pulse rate, associated with profuse sweating. Cardiac irregularities may occur, and lead to death. The usual forms of sedation, such as chlorpromazine, do not affect these bursts of activity, and attempts have been made to reduce their effects by the use of beta-adrenergic blockers, such as propranolol, sometimes combined with bethanidine, to counteract the alpha-adrenergic effects. This régime has met with some success, but great care must be exercised, to avoid sudden hypotension.

Hyperpyrexia

By definition, the 'core' temperature rises above 40°C. It does not often do so with simple infections, and convulsions may occur in children before this level is reached. Associated dehydration may increase the temperature. Damage in the midbrain area may lead to uncontrollable pyrexia as may an abnormal reaction to drugs.

Such a high temperature may in itself cause brain damage, and in some cases the brain 'thermostat' in the hypothalamus may be deranged, so that any fall of temperature will cause shivering until the high temperature is reached again. Oxygen consumption is enormous, and there is always associated hypoxia, especially if convulsions also occur. Acid metabolites rapidly accumulate and death occurs unless treatment is urgently undertaken. Hyperpyrexia occurring as an abnormal response to drugs, has been found to have a familial incidence in some instances. Hypersensitivity occurs usually in response to suxamethonium (a depolarising muscle relaxant) but sometimes to halothane, and occasionally to any other drug.

The onset of pyrexia is rapid, and shivering occurs if the patient is not anaesthetised. The aims of treatment are to lower the body temperature to normal by cooling, to stop muscle activity thereby decreasing heat production, to give oxygen, and to treat metabolic acidosis.

Accordingly the patient is paralysed with a non-depolarising muscle relaxant such as tubocurarine, intubated, and the lungs are artificially ventilated with oxygen. Skin vasodilatation should be encouraged with such drugs as chlorpromazine or droperidol. Intravenous fluids are given, and sodium bicarbonate in dosage calculated from the measured base deficit.

Cooling is achieved by fans, ice-packs, ice baths, or even intragastric iced water. Unless the pyrexia can be controlled rapidly there is a high mortality rate.

Drug Overdosage

The risk of ingestion of harmful substances is well known in childhood. The clinical signs are very variable, depending on the nature of the substance swallowed. Unconsciousness is most likely to be caused by hypnotics such as barbiturates and glutethimide, but may sometimes be associated with aspirin and tranquillizers. Ingestion of kerosene can be associated with inhalation pneumonia, and that of caustic soda with burns to the mouth, oesophagus and trachea. It is helpful if the poison can be identified and the necessary antidote given.

The place of induced vomiting or gastric lavage is debatable. Certainly these are contraindicated in the case of kerosene and caustic materials. If the patient is seen soon after ingestion, vomiting may be induced in the home if the patient is conscious, but apomorphine should be avoided. It is doubtful if gastric lavage is any use with barbiturate after 4 hours have elapsed, but it has been stated always to be of value in aspirin poisoning. If the child is conscious, gastric washout with a large tube is a reasonably safe, if unpleasant procedure. However, with an unconscious patient the danger of inhalation is great, and a cuffed or tightly fitting endotracheal tube should be passed before lavage is undertaken.

If a specific antidote is not available, the patient should be treated symptomatically if convulsions, cardiac failure or arrhythmias occur. Hydration must be maintained, and the unconscious state treated on the usual lines. Active reheating of hypothermic patients should be avoided, unless the temperature is less than 30 °C, when the danger of ventricular fibrillation is great. If the blood pressure is low, vasopressors should be avoided, but plasma expanders may be used. Analeptic drugs are contraindicated as a treatment for respiratory depression; they only increase oxygen demand, and may cause convulsions from cerebral stimulation.

If the metabolism of the drug by the body is low, other means of assisting its elimination may be needed. The methods available are:
  (a) forced diuresis, alkaline or neutral
  (b) peritoneal dialysis
  (c) haemodialysis
  (d) passage of blood over ion exchange resins
  (e) exchange transfusion

The simplest method is that of forced diuresis, provided the drug is excreted by the kidneys, and that these have not been damaged by the poison. Some drugs (e.g. aspirin) are excreted more readily if the urine is alkaline, and sodium bicarbonate is usually used to achieve this. Diuresis is normally obtained with mannitol, and large quantities of intravenous fluids. If the drug is not excreted by the kidney, peritoneal or haemodialysis may be necessary.

Barbiturates

These cause depression of respiration and of metabolism. If unconsciousness is present, it is usually associated with some degree of hypoventilation and hypothermia. Analeptics should be avoided, and artificial ventilation of the lungs undertaken if necessary. Renal excretion may be assisted by forced diuresis, but alkalinisation is of value only with barbitone and phenobarbitone overdosage. Blood levels of the drug should be measured, and used as a guide to the success of treatment.

Aspirin

This drug is especially dangerous in young children, overdosage sometimes occurring inadvertently during aspirin medication. As soon as poisoning is diagnosed, the stomach should be washed out, with due precautions. The mode of presentation varies, according to the age of the patient, and the degree of poisoning. Aspirin causes a mixed disturbance of acid/base metabolism, consisting of a simultaneous respiratory alkalosis, from stimulation of the respiratory centre, and metabolic acidosis resulting from an increased metabolic rate, increased oxygen requirement, ketosis, and circulating salicylate anions.

In mild poisoning in children, the presentation is of hypocapnia and respiratory alkalosis. Most patients under four years of age, and nearly all under one year, present with a metabolic acidosis, and some are unconscious and convulsing. Respiratory depression is unusual, but can occur.

At first the urine is alkaline, and a diuresis occurs. This, associated with vomiting, will deplete potassium, which will favour preferential excretion of hydrogen ions, and the urine becomes acid. Aspirin is not excreted well in an acid urine.

The toxicity of salicylate is determined by the free salicylate level in the serum, and this should be measured as a guide to treatment and its success. The danger level is considered to be higher than 30 mg/100 ml in children.

In all but the mildest poisoning, excretion of salicylate should be assisted by forced alkaline diuresis, especially in young children. Serum electrolyte levels should be estimated frequently.

Drowning

Sometimes immersion may cause reflex cardiac arrest, from laryngeal spasm, or very cold water, and in such instances there will be little water in the lungs. The majority of cases of drowning will be associated with swallowing and inhalation of large quantities of water, and whatever particulate matter happens to be therein. Theoretically there are differences between drowning in fresh and salt water.

Sea water is hypertonic relative to blood, and water is drawn into the alveoli from the vascular compartment. Sodium, magnesium and chloride ions pass into the blood, there is rapid onset of pulmonary oedema and death may follow haemoconcentration and hypovolaemia. Alveolar damage may cause exudation.

Fresh water is hypotonic, and water is transferred to the blood, with resulting haemodilution, haemolysis, hyperkalaemia (due to red cell breakdown) and circulatory overload.

These differences have not been found in practice. Fresh water contains irritant particulate matter causing alveolar damage and is not always hypotonic. Large amounts of water whether salt or fresh act as an alveolar irritant and damage causes loss of protein into the alveoli, irrespective of the direction of electrolyte transfer. The resultant pulmonary oedema decreases the area of alveolar surface available for gas exchange and causes hypoxia and hypovolaemia.

The treatment of drowning depends on the length of immersion and severity of the condition. Water is invariably swallowed, and the stomach should be emptied to avoid the danger of vomiting and inhalation, especially in unconscious patients.

If the patient is conscious early detection of the onset of pulmonary changes is necessary and oxygen should be given if needed. Hypovolaemia should be treated with intravenous plasma.

If the patient is unconscious, or pulmonary damage severe, an endotracheal tube should be passed, the bronchial tree aspirated, and artificial ventilation given as required. Bronchial lavage *may* help to remove particulate matter, but is usually unrewarding. Systemic arterial and central venous pressure will indicate the state of the circulation. Serial serum electrolyte measurements, blood gas estimations and acid/base determinations are necessary. Hypoxia may lead to cerebral damage and this will be related to the length of immersion. Hypothermia will protect the brain to some extent, but some degree of cerebral oedema is inevitable in severe cases. Intravenous 20 per cent mannitol is used to treat this, and oxygenation should be maintained. However, if pulmonary oedema is severe, oxygenation may be poor, and the type of artificial ventilation pattern required, with a high mean intrathoracic pressure, may increase the cerebral oedema. Mortality is high in severe drowning, but prompt attention to the maintenance of the circulation and oxygenation may be successful in the less severe cases.

Diabetes Mellitus

It is seldom necessary to treat either diabetic coma or hypoglycaemic convulsions in an intensive therapy ward, as prompt diagnosis and energetic treatment after admission will result in reasonably rapid improvement in both instances. However if cardiac arrest or irregularities have occurred, intensive care may be needed.

Moreover diabetic ketoacidosis may complicate some other condition necessitating I.T.U. admission.

Knowledge of the diabetic state, and a history of diet, insulin dosage and infection, are important in the differentiation of these conditions. Blood sugar estimation should always be done together with a measurement of the circulating ketones. Hypoglycaemia is characterised by good hydration, a full pulse, normal blood pressure and is readily reversed with an intravenous injection of hypertonic glucose if the patient cannot swallow.

Diabetic coma is associated with dehydration, metabolic acidosis, hyperventilation, an odour of acetone, hyperglycaemia and hyperkalaemia. It is slow in onset, and results from an infection, or gastrointestinal disturbance, or a change in insulin sensitivity.

Treatment with intravenous sodium chloride, sodium bicarbonate, and soluble insulin, should be energetic, but may result in a sudden lowering of the serum potassium level, and this must be checked frequently. Once dehydration and acidosis are controlled, and the blood sugar level reduced to more normal levels, consciousness returns within four to six hours, when fluids should be given by mouth. Infections must be treated appropriately.

CHAPTER

18

Emergency Resuscitation

Sudden death may occur as a result primarily of cardiac arrest or of respiratory arrest, but the two are closely interrelated and it is probably preferable to refer to 'cardio-respiratory arrest'. It is important that both resident medical staff and nursing staff are able to recognise this before death occurs and to institute appropriate treatment. Procrastination and unnecessary delay in commencing resuscitative measures make a successful outcome unlikely. It is therefore mandatory that a well recognised procedure is employed and every member of the intensive therapy unit staff *must* be familiar with the steps to be taken.

Management falls into definite phases—recognition, restoration of function, and post-arrest management. In order that equipment shall be provided as quickly as possible a 'resuscitation trolley' should be available, the contents of which are given at the end of the chapter.

Although 'sudden' arrest is frequently referred to as a catastrophe occurring without warning, in most instances in childhood (apart from inhalation of vomit or adverse reactions to drugs) a careful review of the patient's physical state and other data reveals that premonitory signs were present, neglect of which precipitated the crisis.

RESPIRATORY ARREST

Respiratory inadequacy may be due to a variety of causes:
1. Lack of inspired oxygen.

2. Central depression of respiration; for example, drug overdosage, cerebrovascular accident, cerebral oedema, poliomyelitis, spinal injury in the cervical region.
3. Peripheral interference with ventilation; for example, external compression of the airway, obstruction of the airway (tongue falling back, blood, vomit, foreign bodies etc.), pneumothorax, haemothorax, muscular paralysis or spasm.
4. Impaired gaseous exchange, as in pulmonary oedema.
5. Impaired oxygen transport; for example, shock, cardiac arrest, carbon monoxide poisoning.
6. Impaired cellular respiration, as in cyanide poisoning.

Whatever the *cause* of respiratory inadequacy, the most important consequence is loss of consciousness from hypoxia and hypercarbia, and this can have secondary effects, such as acute respiratory obstruction from falling back of the tongue, or the lack of cough and palatal reflexes may lead to the inhalation of vomit.

Respiratory arrest may follow. When arrest occurs, cyanosis and convulsions will be present within one minute, and an initial tachycardia will be replaced by bradycardia. Within three minutes all respiratory efforts will have ceased, and within five minutes the blood pressure will have fallen to a level incompatible with survival.

In cardio-respiratory resuscitation, measures to *restore respiration* must take precedence, because without adequate oxygenation no treatment of concurrent impairment of cardiac function is likely to be successful. The measures required are in general simple, and are described later.

CARDIAC ARREST

It must be stressed that cardiac arrest is a *clinical diagnosis*. It may be due to asystole, or ventricular fibrillation, or the heart beat may not in fact have ceased but *poor cardiac action* is present, in which case a relatively normal electrocardiographic appearance, albeit with low voltages, may be found. Cardiac arrest is *not* diagnosed by the electrocardiogram; the important feature is the inability of the heart to eject properly, and therefore a state of extreme hypotension and absence of the circulation exists. To wait for an electrocardiogram before instituting resuscitative measures will lead to disaster.

Cardiac arrest may be due to:
1. Vagal slowing of the heart, due to stimulation of the pharyngeal plexus (intubation, laryngoscopy, bronchoscopy).
2. Acute hypoxia; for example, asphyxia, inhalation of vomit.
3. Drug overdosage; for example, potassium chloride given intravenously too quickly and in too great concentration, intravenous cardiac glycosides.
4. Allergy or idiosyncrasy (anaphylactic shock).
5. Cardiac arrhythmias; for example, Stoke-Adams attack.

Anoxia rapidly follows cardiac arrest, leading to loss of consciousness, respiratory arrest and irreversible brain damage. In general terms, the more highly specialised a tissue, the more sensitive it is to oxygen lack.

The diagnosis can be made from the pale, cyanotic appearance, the loss of consciousness, and absence of respiratory effort, the absence of peripheral pulses best estimated by feeling the carotid artery, and the dilated pupils which do not react to light. This does *not* indicate that the patient is beyond help, but *does* mean that restoration of oxygen supply to the tissues, particularly the brain, must be obtained as quickly as possible. Absence of the carotid pulse indicates no ejection or grossly inadequate ejection by the heart, and pupil dilatation, which occurs within forty-five seconds, implies cerebral ischaemia. It is usually reckoned that the brain can withstand only three minutes of anoxia before irreversible damage occurs. This, however, requires some qualification. In patients suffering from chronic hypoxia (e.g. congenital cyanotic heart disease) the brain may be tolerant of slightly longer periods of anoxia (although it is more difficult to resuscitate the heart in such patients, particularly if the anatomical malformation militates against the production of a good output by massage). Moreover, if the patient's body temperature is subnormal this in itself will reduce the oxygen requirements of the brain and confer some protection against acute anoxia.

THE TEAM AND THE PROCEDURE

The nursing staff in an intensive therapy unit are the most likely individuals to be concerned in the recognition of cardio-respiratory arrest. At least two nurses should be available in order to begin resuscitation and the treatment must be carried out in an orderly logical manner. Two alarms are necessary; the first is an internal alarm within the unit, which must be capable of activation from each bed side station, and probably an audible alarm is best. The second alarm is via the hospital's telephone system, whereby, if a certain priority number is dialled (for example 222), the hospital telephone exchange is alerted, and the medical members of the resuscitation team (the duty I.T.U. registrar and the duty anaesthetist) are notified.

On diagnosing cardio-respiratory arrest the nurse concerned rings the alarm bell to summon the second nurse and if possible a third. She immediately makes sure that the upper airway is clear, aspirating vomit if necessary, and then commences artificial ventilation with a face mask and rebreathing bag receiving 100 per cent oxygen. *This is all that she can effectively do unaided*; if assistance is slow in coming, she *may* have to carry out mouth to mouth breathing and external cardiac massage, but it is very difficult for one person to perform both of these manoeuvres effectively.

The second nurse commences external cardiac massage, while the third nurse alerts the telephone exchange and wheels the resuscitation trolley to the bed side.

The method of performing external cardiac massage depends on the size of the child. With a baby effective massage can be done by placing the left hand behind the thorax, and compressing the sternum backwards, *with the fingers* of the right hand, in a rhythmical manner towards the spine. With toddlers and older children a firm surface behind the thorax is essential, and a suitable board is placed underneath the patient. In the toddler the heel of one hand is used to compress the sternum, but in the older child, with a more rigid chest, it may be necessary to place one hand on top of the other and compress the sternum with both. Excessive force is never necessary and may fracture ribs. *At this stage time should not be taken to connect an electrocardiographic oscilloscope to the patient.* At all ages time must be allowed for the heart to fill so that a rate exceeding 70/minute is not practical and indeed interferes with adequate pulmonary ventilation. The heart must be compressed sufficiently forcibly to produce a palpable pulse, preferably felt in the femoral artery. Palpation of the carotid pulse may be misleading; it must be appreciated that external cardiac massage empties the ventricles into the aorta and pulmonary

Emergency Resuscitation

artery, but it also empties the right atrium into the great veins, so that a venous wave can be felt in the neck. If this is thought to be a carotid artery pulse, one may think adequate cerebral perfusion is being achieved when in fact the cardiac output may be very low. Unfortunately external cardiac massage does *not* act as a method of artificial respiration, so that ventilation with oxygen using a rebreathing bag must be continued.

When the medical team arrives the first priority is to obtain more efficient pulmonary ventilation, which necessitates the passage of an oral endotracheal tube. If necessary a tube is passed to deflate the stomach. External cardiac massage is continued, and if an intravenous infusion is not already running one is set up without delay. The patient is connected via standard limb leads to an E.C.G. oscilloscope and the rhythm is inspected. Interruption of the cardiac massage for a few seconds from time to time will enable one to see whether a normal electrocardiogram is being obtained, and whether a good systemic pressure is being achieved without assistance. *A regularly occurring complex does not necessarily mean an adequate cardiac output.* At this stage the possibilities are:

1. Normal sinus rhythm is present with a good cardiac output.

2. A regular cardiac cycle is present, but with delayed conduction, with QRS complexes and S–T segment changes of hypoxia, while the blood pressure is low.

3. An arrhythmia is present, perhaps runs of ventricular premature contractions, or ventricular tachycardia, both with low cardiac output; or ventricular fibrillation with no output.

4. Complete asystole (a straight line electrocardiogram).

In the first instance the immediate problem is obviously over, *although the cause of the arrest must be sought and corrected.*

In the second, third and fourth cases an attempt must be made to improve cardiac action. In every instance of cardio-respiratory arrest poor tissue perfusion (even with cardiac massage) results in a metabolic acidosis, and at least a partial correction of this should be effected by giving intravenous 8·4 per cent sodium bicarbonate solution according to the formula in Chapter 5 on an estimated base deficit of 10–20 mEq/L depending on the length of time of inadequate circulation. Further bicarbonate may be necessary, and is given after acid/base biochemical measurement. It is important to realise that intravenous sodium bicarbonate has a very high pH and is injurious to tissues; perivenous leakage is likely to be followed by necrosis of superficial tissues, so that it is preferable to give the injections by 'shot' into the intravenous infusion, and to make sure that no concentrated solution remains in the peripheral veins by washing through with normal saline. It is advisable *not* to attempt intracardiac injections using sodium bicarbonate.

Correction of a base deficit may cause improvement in the second instance above, or cardiac output may be increased by careful intravenous injection of calcium chloride 10 per cent, and/or adrenaline 1:10,000 solution given in small amounts to a total of 1 mg.

When arrhythmias are present, such as ventricular premature contractions or ventricular tachycardia. the use of adrenaline is contraindicated and is dangerous. However, if a fine ventricular fibrillation is found, the use of adrenaline will often convert this into a coarse one which will respond more readily to electrical defibrillation.

The treatment of a patient with complete asystole is difficult. In these cases venous filling of the heart is often very poor and intravenous injections are unlikely to reach the heart in time and in adequate concentration. Under these circumstances intracardiac injections, while not advisable as a general rule, should be tried. The safest route is to insert a long needle, mounted on the syringe, to the left of the xiphisternum and to pass it upwards, backwards and to the right. This will then enter the right ventricle, and injury to coronary vessels or the lung is unlikely to occur. Adrenaline and calcium chloride can be given by this route.

Ventricular fibrillation only rarely reverts to normal rhythm with massage alone. The hypoxic, acidotic heart is difficult, if not impossible to defibrillate, so adequate oxygenation, the administration of bicarbonate, and cardiac massage to obtain a good coronary blood flow must precede attempts at electrical defibrillation.

Defibrillation is best achieved by the passage of a *direct* current through the chest and therefore through the heart from an electrical defibrillator, for a period of 2–4 milliseconds. The quantity of electrical energy that can be used can be varied. Electrodes liberally smeared with electrode jelly, are firmly applied to either side of the chest, and a shock is given according to the child's size, all assistants standing clear of the child while the shock is given. It is best to begin with a shock of 20 joules and to increase if necessary to a maximum of 200 joules.

Emergency Resuscitation

Defibrillation is most effective when the myocardium is in a state of coarse fibrillation; a very fine fibrillation rarely responds to D.C. shock and should first be converted to coarse fibrillation by adrenaline and the continuation of external cardiac massage.

Successful defibrillation may result in restoration of a relatively normal sinus rhythm, or cardiac asystole. Even if sinus rhythm is restored, *if the cardiac output is poor external cardiac massage must be continued* until effective cardiac contractions are obtained.

Following restoration of a good heart beat spontaneous respiration may or may not be resumed. *Ventilation must be effective* and inadequate respiration must be treated by continuing artificial ventilation of the lungs. At this stage the oral tube may be changed for a nasotracheal tube for ease of management. *Inadequate breathing is not an indication to use nikethamide or other analeptic drugs* which cannot stimulate the respiratory centre if this is suffering from the results of hypoxia, but may provoke the onset of cerebral convulsions.

If a good cardiac output is not achieved by resuscitative measures, a decision must be made as to the length of time these are to be continued. It is wise to reassess the patient every 20 minutes. A very poor circulation with fixed dilated pupils is an ominous sign. It must be emphasised that the decision to stop resuscitation is one to be made by the medical and not the nursing staff.

POST CARDIO-RESPIRATORY ARREST MANAGEMENT

After the acute crisis has been dealt with, further investigations may be necessary to determine the cause of the arrest, and this corrected if possible.

Post-arrest management is directed towards the support of those systems which have been, or may have been, affected by the period of poor circulation and hypoxia. In order of importance these are the nervous system, the kidneys and the heart itself.

Nervous tissue is very sensitive to oxygen lack, the degree of damage being directly related to the degree of specialisation of the nerve cells concerned. Thus the higher centres are much more susceptible to a relatively short period of hypoxia than are the lower centres, and not uncommonly after a period of cardio-respiratory resuscitation the patient remains unconscious for a varying length of time, the duration of which depends on the insult to the cerebral cortex. Severe brain damage will be revealed by profound unconsciousness, fixed dilated pupils with papilloedema, and a spastic decerebrate type of rigidity. Less severe damage may be followed by convulsions, requiring the management outlined in Chapter 17. Apneustic, gasping type of breathing is an ominous sign, almost always indicating a fatal outcome, while Cheyne-Stokes breathing, although serious, does not necessarily have a bad prognosis. Much of the neurological picture may be due to cerebral oedema, itself secondary to brain damage, and a decision will have to be made whether or not to use osmotic diuretics such as mannitol in an attempt to *prevent* serious oedema occurring. It is doubtful if the promotion of a diuresis will do much to affect severe oedema. It is however, important *not* to use such therapy until one is sure that renal function has not been impaired, otherwise an expansion of the vascular compartment will occur possibly resulting in cardiac overload. A suitable dose of mannitol is 1 gm/Kg of bodyweight given intravenously.

Damage in the region of the midbrain not infrequently results in disturbances of the body temperature-regulating mechanism, so that hyperpyrexia occurs. While the treatment of the brain damage *without* hyperpyrexia by means of surface cooling to produce a moderate degree of hypothermia (e.g. 35 °C) is somewhat controversial, the use of cooling to lower the temperature of the hyperpyretic patient is essential. Hyperpyrexia if uncontrolled is invariably fatal, and even non-fatal elevations of body temperature increase the metabolic rate and therefore oxygen requirements. Surface cooling can be by ice packs applied to the trunk (crushed ice in thick polythene bags is preferable), and by cooling fans, the body being completely exposed. Overcooling is to be avoided, as this results in vasoconstriction in the limbs with the production of metabolic acidosis, and excessive cooling will result in cardiac arrest. It is also obviously difficult to achieve satisfactory cooling in a restless patient who is generating heat by muscular activity.

Vasodilatation to increase heat loss is helpful and may be achieved by such drugs as chlorpromazine or droperidol. If these measures are ineffective in controlling pyrexia, a muscle relaxant should be given and the lungs ventilated.

Renal function may be normal after the arrest but in all cases it is advisable to measure urinary excretion accurately using an indwelling catheter, and to record both volume and specific gravity. Complete renal shut-down may follow hypoxia, and may last for a varying period of time, during which the blood urea and serum potassium levels must be estimated repeatedly in order to decide if dialysis is required. A prolonged period of renal hypotension may result in acute tubular necrosis with initial anuria and the possibility in the recovery phase of failure to conserve body water, with the passage of large volumes of dilute urine and a loss of considerable quantities of electrolytes.

The heart itself is placed third in order of priority in post-arrest care because, if the myocardium is healthy, with no anatomical abnormalities, it is remarkably tolerant of a period of hypoxia. This is in contradistinction to cardiac arrest in the presence of a severe cardiac anomaly in which case resuscitation is difficult to achieve and may be followed by further episodes of arrest.

Attention must be paid in the post-arrest period to acid/base balance; a metabolic acidosis may persist for a time, necessitating the use of intravenous sodium bicarbonate, and also perhaps measures to improve cardiac output and tissue perfusion, for example, the correction of hypovolaemia.

It must be reiterated that successful resuscitation depends on early diagnosis and effectively applied measures. Not every patient will be saved, and not all will be restored to full function of all systems. Difficulty may be experienced in deciding how long to maintain supportive therapy (artificial ventilation, the use of vasopressor drugs etc.) in a patient who remains profoundly unconscious and unresponsive. It is important to have an electroencephalogram recorded if possible within two hours of the arrest, and repeated at daily intervals thereafter as indicated. A complete absence of cerebral activity with a confident diagnosis of 'cerebral death' should lead to the discontinuing of artificial ventilation of the lungs. This *must* be a medical decision made by more than one consultant.

Finally it should be emphasized that there are certain patients in whom *resuscitation should not be commenced,* for example, a patient with advanced incurable malignant disease. Again, the decision not to employ resuscitation in the event of cardio-respiratory arrest occurring must be made *beforehand* by the consultant in charge of the patient; nursing and junior medical staff cannot be expected to make this decision in the absence of prior instructions. Cardio-respiratory arrest in some patients is a welcome end to incurable suffering.

THE RESUSCITATION TROLLEY

In the I.T.U. environment this does not need to contain drugs, or intravenous equipment (as might perhaps be the case with a trolley designed for ordinary ward use), but the essential apparatus necessary to ventilate the patient and clear the airway, perhaps under direct vision, should be available by the bed. It is convenient for the trolley to have a working surface on which an infant can be placed, older children being dealt with on the cot or bed. The trolley must contain the following in easily accessible compartments:

1. Laryngoscopes of the required sizes, with spare bulbs and batteries.
2. Bronchoscopes with spare light carriers and suction tubes of appropriate size, two suction tubes being available for each bronchoscope in case of blockage.
3. Orotracheal tubes of varying size with connectors and a catheter mount.
4. Guedel airways.
5. Tape etc. for anchoring orotracheal tubes.

Appendix

Doses of drugs commonly used in the I.T.U.

In adults, the doses of drugs commonly used tend to be standard, and often not varied according to the size of the patient. However, such a method cannot be used with the wide range of size in childhood. Accurate prescribing of drugs is essential.

Drug dosage is most accurately related to body surface area. If prescribing is done on a body weight basis, the younger patients will receive a low dosage, as they have a relatively larger surface area.

However, surface area is not often measured, whereas weight always is. A rough estimate can be used as follows:

at 10 Kg give 25 per cent of adult dose
14 Kg give 33 per cent of adult dose
22 Kg give 50 per cent of adult dose
36 Kg give 70 per cent of adult dose.

With many of the drugs used in intensive care, proportional underdosing in young children is not of great importance, and the dose can be conveniently remembered in mg/Kg. In the following dosage guide, the dose in mg/Kg for infants is given, also the normal adult dose, so the required dose can readily be estimated.

Drug dosage should never be made on age alone, as there can be a great range of body weight, especially in intensive care, when many of the children are small for age. Patients in some age-groups are hyper-sensitive to certain drugs—e.g. neonates are very sensitive to curare-like drugs, and dosage should be cautious; children under one year tend to be readily depressed by morphine-like drugs, and the dose should be reduced.

Drugs which are given routinely are administered at regularly spaced intervals during the 24 hours. Those drugs which are given to control acute conditions, such as muscle relaxants, analgesics, vasodilators and anti-epileptics, are given as necessary without regard to time interval, and preferably intravenously. The possibility of side-effects must be anticipated, and provision made to deal with them.

Appendix

Drug	Mode of Action	Route	Frequency	Dose Infants	Dose Adults	Comments
Adrenaline 1:1,000	α & β adrenergic effects	I.V.		1–25 mg/500 ml as required, diluted		To improve cardiac output. Danger of arrhythmia, tachycardia, vasoconstriction
Alcuronium	Muscle relaxant	I.V. or I.M.	as required	0.2 mg/Kg	10–15 mg	To control patient on ventilator
Aminophylline	Bronchodilator	oral or I.M.	6–8 hourly	2.5 mg/Kg	100 mg	Slow I.V. injection. Painful I.M.
Atropine Sulphate	Anticholinergic	S.C. or I.V.	once	0.015 mg/Kg	up to 0.6 mg	Loss of sweating may cause pyrexia in babies
Calcium Chloride 10%	1gm = 9 mEq Ca^{++}	oral I.V.	6–8 hourly once	50 mg/Kg diluted, dose calculated from deficit	2 gm	For hypocalcaemia. Improves myocardial contractility. Very irritant to tissues
Calcium gluconate 10%	1gm = 4.5 mEq Ca^{++}	oral I.V.	6–8 hourly once	100 mg/Kg 30 mg/Kg, diluted, slowly	4 gm	Slower effect than chloride, not so irritant
Chloral hydrate	Hypnotic	oral	8 hourly	30 mg/Kg	1.5 gm	
Chlorothiazide	Diuretic	oral	once daily	125 mg/Kg	1 gm	Depletes body potassium
Chlorpromazine	Tranquillizer α adrenergic blocker	oral or I.M. I.M. or I.V.	6 hourly as required	1 mg/Kg 5 mg repeated as needed	50 mg	

Drug	Mode of Action	Route	Frequency	Dose Infants	Dose Adults	Comments
Diazepam	Tranquilliser Anticonvulsant	oral or I.M. I.M. or I.V.	8 hourly as required	0.3 mg/Kg up to 1 mg/Kg	5 to 10 mg	May cause gastritis in repeated dosage. Painful I.V. injection
Digoxin	Cardiac glycoside	oral I.M. or I.V.	8– 12 hourly	0.006 mg/Kg 0.003 mg/Kg	0.25 mg 0.125 mg	For rapid digitalisation— 6 × stated dose once, then 2 × stated dose at 6 hours and 12 hours
Diprophylline	Bronchodilator	oral, I.M. or I.V.	8 hourly	5 mg/Kg	200 mg	
Droperidol	Tranquilliser α adrenergic blocker	oral, I.M. or I.V.	8 hourly as required	0.2–0.6 mg/Kg increments of 2.5 or 5 mg	5–15 mg	May cause oculogyric crises in large dosage
Frusemide	Diuretic	oral I.M. or I.V.	alt. days or once daily	2 mg/Kg 1 mg/Kg	80 mg 40 mg	Depletes body potassium
Heparin	Anticoagulant	I.V.		3 mg/Kg	3 mg/Kg	1 mg ≃ 100 units. Repeat according to clotting time
Isoprenaline	β adrenergic effects	I.V.	As required, diluted 1–25 mg/500 ml			May cause tachycardia and ventricular arrhythmias
Lignocaine	For control of arrhythmias	I.V.	intermittent infusion	1–2 mg/Kg 1 gm/200 ml as required		

Drug	Mode of Action	Route	Frequency	Dose Infants	Dose Adults	Comments
Morphine	Narcotic analgesic	I.M.	as required	avoid	10 mg	Antidote—nalorphine
Nalorphine	Antidote for narcotic overdose	I.M. or I.V.	as required	0.2 mg/Kg	10 mg	May cause respiratory depression in overdose
Pancuronium	Muscle relaxant	I.M. or I.V.	as required	0.1 mg/Kg	4–6 mg	To control patient on ventilator
Papaveretum	Narcotic analgesic	I.M.	as required	avoid	15 mg	Smaller dose I.V. Antidote—nalorphine
Phenoperidine	Narcotic analgesic respiratory depressant	S.C. or I.V. S.C. or I.V.	as required	avoid 0.1 mg/Kg	0.5–1 mg 2–4 mg	Use larger dose only when patient on ventilator. Antidote—nalorphine
Phenoxybenzamine	α adrenergic blocker	I.V.	once	1 mg/Kg diluted and given over 1 hour		Effect lasts 24–48 hours. Take care to maintain CVP with fluids I.V.
Phenytoin	Anticonvulsant Antiarrhythmic	oral I.V.	8 hourly as required	2.5 mg/Kg 1.5 mg/Kg	100 mg 100 mg	
Potassium chloride	1 gm KCL = 13 mEq K⁺	oral I.V.	6–8 hourly see Chapter 4	50 ng/Kg	2 gm	Give only in presence of urine output. Stat doses I.V. may cause cardiac arrest
Propranolol	β adrenergic blocker	oral I.V.	8 hourly as required	0.5 mg/Kg —	20 mg 10 mg	Caution with I.V. injection—may cause hypotension and bronchospasm

Drug	Mode of Action	Route	Frequency	Dose Infants	Dose Adults	Comments
Protamine sulphate	Antidote for heparin	I.V.	Slowly, 1 mg for each 100 units heparin			
Reserpine	Hypotensive agent	oral I.V. or I.M.	once or 8 hourly	0.012 mg/Kg 0.07 mg/Kg	0.5 mg 2.5 mg	Side effect—depression
Spironolactone	Diuretic	oral	8 hourly	0.6 mg/Kg	25 mg	
Thiopentone sodium 2.5%	Induction of anaesthesia	I.V.	once	4–8 mg/Kg		Causes respiratory depression. May be used to control convulsions
Thymoxamine	α adrenergic blocker	I.V.	as required	0.1 mg/Kg		Effect lasts about 4 hours
Tubocurarine	Muscle relaxant	I.V. or I.M.	as required	0.5 mg/Kg	25–30 mg	To control patient on ventilator
STEROIDS Hydrocortisone hemisuccinate		I.M. or I.V.	6 hourly	50 mg	100 mg	50–150 mg/kg in single dose I.V. to cause vasodilatation in shock
Dexamethasone		I.V.	single	6 mg/Kg		Single dose for vasodilatation in shock
Prednisolone		oral	8–12 hourly	0.7 mg/Kg	30 mg	For maintenance therapy

Index

Acetyl
  choline 85
  cysteine 151
Acid, aspiration syndrome of Mendelson 165, 229
Acid/base balance 51
  correction of disturbed 57
  determinations 142
  disturbances 52
Acidosis 48, 76, 205, 211
  effect on cardiac output 76
  lactic 46, 186
  metabolic 51, 52, 57, 185, 191
  renal 'shut down' in 191
  respiratory, 48, 52, 196
Adrenaline 85, 86
  blockers 86
Aerosols 116, 151
Air bronchogram 106, 129
'Air' embolism 197, 198
Airway
  artificial 140, 153, 159
  aspiration of 141, 160
  Guedel 146, 232
  in unconscious patient 232
  resistance 171
Alarm, warning 248
Alcuronium 162
Aldosterone 23, 204

Alkalosis 48
  and low potassium 191
  metabolic 26, 35, 52, 186, 191, 205
  respiratory 48, 52
Alveolar gas constituents 60
  unit 170
Amino-acids, essential 37
Aminophylline 165
'Aminosol' infusions 39–46, 211
Ammonium chloride 35
Anaemia, in renal failure 205, 211
Analgesics 171
Anoxia 69
Antidiuretic hormone 23, 24, 200, 204
Anuria 201, 207
Aortic bodies 61
  stenosis 181
Aorto-pulmonary shunt 230
APGAR score 219
Apneustic breathing 252
Apnoea monitor 103, 143, 223
Arrest, cardiac 246
  cardio-respiratory 245
  respiratory 245
Arrhythmias, cardiac 192, 211, 249
Arterial cannulation 94, 95, 142
  system 78

Arteritis, necrotizing 194
Artificial airway 140, 153
  management 159
Artificial nose 114
Asphyxia, of newborn 226
Aspiration, of trachea 141, 160
Aspirin 242
Asthma 131, 148, 164
Astrup 50, 53, 145, 149
Atelectasis, with high oxygen concentrations 69
  miliary 195
  postoperative 129, 172
Atresia, of bile ducts 230
  of oesophagus 278
Atrial septostomy 230
Azotaemia 200, 204

Balloon septostomy 230
Barbiturates 241
Barnet ventilator 118
Beta-adrenergic blockade 194, 239
Bethanidine 212, 239
Bicarbonate, depletion 57
  in newborn 225
  standard 50
Bile ducts, atresia of 230
Bilirubin 230
Bird ventilator 119
Bladder, care of 136
Blalock-Hanlon operation 230
Bleeding, intra-thoracic 178
  in renal failure 205
  post by-pass 187
Blood, buffer systems 49
  culture 17, 149
  distribution to tissues 89
  flow 87
  gas studies 142, 149
  gas transport 66
  pressure, measurement of 93
  pressure, systemic 76–8, 93–5, 143
  replacement 189, 226
  transfusion 187, 191
  urea 204, 206

vessels 89
  volume, increased 182
  volume, low 189
  volume, measurement of 30
  warming coil 226
Bourns ventilator 123
Bronchial, drainage 171
  lavage 152, 174, 229
  obstruction 114
Bronchiolitis 131, 148, 168
Bronchoscopy 177
Bronchospasm 149
Bronchogram, 'air' 106, 129, 167
Buffer systems 48–50
Bundle, atrio-ventricular of His 84
Burns 200
Bypass, cardio-pulmonary 183, 184

Calcium 28–30, 191, 228
  chloride 250
  gluconate 191
Calorie 36
  requirements 38
Calorific food values 37
Candida albicans 222
Cannula, arterial 94
  in neonate 223
  management of 142
  venous 96
Capacitance vessels 89
Capillaries 89
Capillary sphincters 89
Carbamino-haemoglobin 67
Carbohydrates, in diet 37
Carbon dioxide 67
  combining power 35
  dissociation curve 68
  retention 72
  transport 51, 67
Carbonic anhydrase 49
Cardiac, arrest 206
  failure 23, 206
  filling pressure 75
  massage 248

Index

Cardiac—*cont.*
  output   73–4, 99, 188
  output and lungs   81
  ouput, maintenance of   188
  tamponade   190
  work   76
Cardio-pulmonary bypass   184
  cardiac failure after   191
  fluids after   197
  metabolic effects   186
  monitoring after   186
Cardio-respiratory arrest   145, 246
Cardioscope   143
Cardiovascular centres   84
Carotid bodies   61
Catecholamines   85–7, 186, 193
Catheter, urinary   136
Central venous pressure   75, 79, 95–7, 142, 143, 181, 189
Centre, cardio-inhibitor   85
  cardio-stimulator   85
  pneumotaxic   61
  respiratory   61
Charting of data   143
Chemoreceptors   61, 85
Chest drainage, management   139
Cheyne-Stokes breathing   252
'Chironseal' bag   224
Chloride, ammonium   35
  ion   25
  shift   25, 51
Chronotropic effect   86
Chylothorax   129
Cilia   114
Circulation, in newborn   82
Clark electrode   56
Coagulation defects   186
Coarctation of aorta   181
  postoperative rebound hypertension   194
Coma   235–6
Compliance, of lung   63, 132, 171
  of ventricle   75
  reduced   132, 171, 181
Conducting system of heart   83
Congenital cardiovascular disease   180–3

Congenital laryngeal stridor   152
Conscious level   102
Consolidation, pulmonary   129
Constant infusion pump   138
Continuous positive pressure breathing   163
Contrast medium   128
Contusion, of lung   179
Convulsions, causes of   236
  in newborn   227
  in water intoxication   24, 206
Convulsive states   236
Corneal ulceration   136, 235
Coronary artery blood flow   76
Creatinine   204
Cross infection   7, 15, 18
'Cut-down' intravenous cannulation   137
Cyanosis   71, 148, 170
Cycling, ventilator, mixed   111
  patient   112
  pressure   111, 112, 113
  time   110, 112
  volume   110, 112, 113

Data presentation   142–3
Dead space   64
  alveolar   65, 170
  anatomical   64, 170
  physiological   65, 170
  total   170
Dead space: tidal volume ratio   170
Defibrillation   192, 250
Dehydration   31
  hypernatraemic   32
  hyponatraemic   32
  isotonic   32
  weight recording in   32
Dextrans, intravenous   194
Diabetes mellitus   244
Diabetic coma, electrolyte imbalance in   24, 26
Dialysis, indications for   212
  peritoneal   213
  problems of   216

Diaphragm, hernia of 133, 229
  splinting of 229
Diarrhoea, fluid loss in 138
Diazepam 162, 237
Diffusion of gases 65
Digitalization 192
Digitalis toxicity, potassium and 192
Diprophylline 168
Dissociation curve, carbon dioxide 68
  oxygen 66
Diuresis, forced 241
  osmotic 208
Diuretics 233
Divider, minute volume 118
Drainage, pericardial 190
  pleural 139, 175, 223
Drew technique 188
Droperidol 161
Drowning 242
Drug administration by nebuliser 116, 151
Dyspnoea 181

Effusion, pleural 129, 150
Eisenmenger state 182
Electric blanket, interference from 98
Electrocardiogram 97, 146
  abnormalities of 99, 100
  artefacts in 97
  in hyperkalaemia 28
  in hypokalaemia 27
Electroencephalogram 102, 253
Electrolyte, balance 225
  disturbances and convulsions 238
  disturbances and the heart 26–8, 76, 191
  in body fluids 33
  infusion solutions 34
Emphysema, surgical 177
Endotracheal intubation, complications of 154–5
  prolonged 154

Endotracheal suction 152
Endotracheal tube 140, 155
  fixation of 154
  length of 129, 155
  size of 154
Energy, of food 36
  requirements 37
Engström ventilator 123, 161
Enzymes, fibrinolytic 179
Ephedrine 165
Epiglottitis 149, 166
Epsilon-aminocaproic acid 187
Ethylene oxide 20
Exercise, heart rate and 78
  pulmonary blood flow and 61, 81, 169
  venous return and 79
Expiratory, phase, of ventilator 111
  resistance 111
External cardiac massage 146
Extracellular fluid 30, 204
Eyes, care of 136, 235

Failure, cardiac 23, 206
  postrenal 201
  prerenal 199
  renal 199
  renal parenchymal 201
Fallot, tetralogy of 182, 230
Fat, brown 221
  in diet 37
  intravenous 39
Fatty acids, essential 37
$F.E.V_1$ 64
Fibrillation, atrial 75, 99
  ventricular 99, 192, 250
Fibrinolysins 187
Fibrinolytic enzymes 179
Fibroplasia, retrolental 69, 221
Fixation, of artificial airway 140, 154, 158
Flow, along tubes 87
Flow generators 109
Fluid, balance 137, 197
  balance, recording 138

Index

Fluid—*cont.*
　exchange in tissues　89
　extracellular　30, 204
　Newtonian　87
　requirement, basic　210
Flutter, atrial　99
Foetal circulation　82
Frusemide　232
Functional residual capacity　64

Galactosaemia　230
Gas injector　110
Gastric, aspirate　138
　dilatation, acute　234
Gastrostomy　234
Generator, flow　109
　pressure　109
　sine wave　109
Glenn operation　194
Glomerular filtration rate　200
Glomerulonephritis　203, 207
Guedel airway　146, 232
Guillain-Barré syndrome　150

Haematocrit　30, 226
Haematological changes, in cardiopulmonary bypass　186
Haemodilution, in cardiopulmonary bypass　185
Haemoglobin　49
　oxygen dissociation curve　66
Haemolysis　202
Haemolytic-uraemic syndrome　203, 207
Haemorrhage, intrathoracic　178
Heart, block　98, 101, 191
　disease, congenital　181, 230
　rate　74, 84–5, 99
　rate, variation of　75
　sounds, splitting of　74
Henderson—Hasselbalch equation　50
Hepatitis　230
Hernia, diaphragmatic　229
His, bundle of　84

Hormone, antidiuretic　200, 204
　parathyroid　29
Humidification　114, 140, 151, 154, 172, 220
Humidifier, artificial nose　114
　nebuliser, gas-driven　115
　nebuliser, ultrasonic　115
　water-bath　116
Hyaline membranes　106, 132
'Hycal'　210
Hydration　233
Hydrocortisone　151
Hydrogen ion concentration　47
Hydrometer　208
Hydronephrosis　207, 209
Hypercarbia　62, 246
Hypercatabolic state　207, 210
Hyperkalaemia　28, 101, 204
　treatment of　36, 211
Hypernatraemia　24
Hypernatraemic dehydration　32
Hyperpyrexia　144, 188, 197, 239, 252
　in neonate　218
　treatment of　240
Hypertension, in renal failure　206, 212
　pulmonary　182
　rebound　194
Hyperventilation　233
Hypocalcaemia　218, 228, 238
Hypocapnia　242
Hypoglycaemia　218, 227, 237
Hypokalaemia　27, 101
Hypomagnesaemia　228
Hyponatraemia　23, 204, 206, 210, 238
Hyponatraemic dehydration　32
Hypoplasia, pulmonary　229
　renal　204
Hypothalamus, temperature control　84, 118, 239
Hypothermia　144, 183
　in brain damage　252
　in neonate　218
　profound　187
　with drug overdosage　241

Hypothyroidism 230
Hypovolaemia 189, 190
Hypoxaemia 69
Hypoxia 69–72, 150, 152, 237
  causes of 71
  chronic 182
  ECG changes 101

I:E ratio 106
Incubator, use of 135, 221
  servo-controlled 144, 221
Incompatibility, A-B-O 230
  Rhesus 230
  transfusion 202
Infant, respiratory physiology 68
  temperature control 104
Infarction, renal 203
Infection, monilia 15
Infra-red lamp 8, 146, 223
Infundibular spasm 182, 194
Injector 109, 118, 119, 122
Inotropic effect 86
Inspiratory, phase, of ventilator 108
Insulin, and sodium pump 24
  glucose and potassium 26
  in diabetic coma 244
  in hyperkalaemia 36, 211
Intensive therapy unit, bed allocation 2, 5
  cross infection 7, 15, 18
  engineering services 11
  equipment 9
  lighting 9
  location 6
  oxygen supply 11
  power supply 12
  rooms in 9
  staffing 6
  vacuum supply 11
  ventilation 12
  warning alarm 14, 248
Intercostal drainage 175
Internal jugular vein catheterization 96
Intracardiac injection 250

'Intralipid' 39, 211, 226
Intrathoracic bleeding 178
Intravenous fluids 34, 138
Intubation, endotracheal 153–4
  nasotracheal 154
Involution, of pulmonary arteries 83, 182
I.P.P.R. 160, 179
Isoprenaline 86–7, 151, 165, 191, 193
Isovolumetric contraction 73

Jackson-Rees tube 155
Jaundice 218, 230

Kernicterus 230

Lactate, sodium 35
Lactic acid 51, 57, 186
Lactic acidosis 46
Laryngeal, oedema 140, 154
  obstruction 131
  stenosis 154, 156
  stridor 151
  web 151
Laryngotracheobronchitis 151, 166
Lignocaine 192
Loosco ventilator 116
Lung, atelectasis 129
  consolidation 129
  distribution of air and blood 61, 64, 81, 169
  'dummy' 112
  rupture 108, 132, 161, 229
  volumes 63

Magnesium 28–30, 225
Mannitol 35, 208–9, 233, 252
Manometer, saline 96
Massage, cardiac 248
Mean intrathoracic pressure 108
Mendelson syndrome 151, 165

Index

Mephanesin 239
Metabolic balance 36–38
Metabolism, anaerobic 51
  of glucose 50
Microcirculation 87, 89, 191
Minute volume 64
Minute volume divider 118
Monilia 15, 17, 218, 222
Monitor, apnoea 103, 223
Monitoring 91
  after cardio-pulmonary bypass 189
  arterial pressure 94
  cannulae 142
  central venous pressure 95
  equipment 8
  in paediatric I.T.U. 92
  nervous system 102
  temperature 104
  tissue perfusion 101
  ventilation 103, 106
Moro reflex 227
Muscle relaxants 161, 237
Mustard operation 194
Myasthenia gravis 150
Myocardial contractility 76

Narcotic analgesics 161
Nasal septum ulceration 140, 155
Nasogastric tube, insertion of 137, 174, 224
  position of 128, 137
Nebuliser, gas driven 115
  ultrasonic 115, 220
Necrosis, tubular 200
Neonate, acid/base balance 225
  blood transfusion 226
  circulation of blood 83
  fluid requirement 22, 225
  general management of 223
  intravenous infusions 137, 225
  neurological state 226
  respiration 219
  risks to 218
  temperature regulation 218
  tetanus in 238

Nephrotic syndrome 200
Nerve, cardio-accelerator 85
Neuritis, peripheral 150
Newtonian fluid 87
Nikethamide 153
Nitrogen, requirement 37
Nodal rhythm 84
Node, atrio-ventricular 84
  sino-atrial 83
Nor-adrenaline 85, 86
Nursing, care 135
  responsibility in emergency 145
Nutrition, in renal failure 210
  parenteral 38

Obstruction, bronchial 114
  in circulation 180
  respiratory 151
Oedema, cerebral 233, 252
  peripheral venous 182
  pulmonary 108, 131, 160, 181, 243
Oesophageal stethoscope 101
Oesophagus, congenital abnormalities of 128, 133, 228
Oliguria 197
  in acute tubular necrosis 202
  in prerenal failure 200
Opisthotonus 148, 238
Orciprenaline 151, 165
Oscilloscope 93, 142
Oscillotonometer 94
Osmolality 208
Osmometer, freezing-point 208
Overdosage, of drugs 240
Oxygen, consumption in convulsions 237
  effects of high concentrations 69, 105, 132, 152, 221
  saturation 66
  tents 152
  therapy 172
  transport 66, 171
Oxygenator, Kay-Cross 184
  Mayo-Gibbon 184
  Rygg 184

Oxygenator—*cont.*
  Temptrol 184
Overhydration 209

Pacemaker, artificial 191–2
  sino-atrial node 83
Pancuronium 162
Papilloedema 252
Paradoxical respiration 175, 223
Paraldehyde 237
Parathyroid hormone 29
Parenteral, fluid 137
  nutrition 38–46
Partial pressure of gas 48
P_{CO_2} 48, 149, 225
  measurement 53
Perfusion, pressure 77
  tissue 89, 101
Peripheral neuritis 150
Peripheral vascular resistance 78, 89
Persistent ductus arteriosus 183
pH 47, 53
Phase, expiratory, of ventilator 111
  inspiratory, of ventilator 108
Phenobarbitone 237
Phenoperidine 161
Phenoxybenzamine 193
Phentolamine 86
Phenytoin 192, 237
Physiotherapy 136, 152, 162, 173, 235
Pierre-Robin syndrome 151–2
Platelet depletion 187
Plethysmograph 103
Pleura 62
Pleural fluid 129, 175
Pleuro-peritoneal hernia 229
Pneumoperitoneum 127
Pneumotachygraph 103, 107
Pneumotaxic centre 61
Pneumothorax 108, 127, 131, 139, 150
  tension 175, 229
P_{O_2}, measurement 55

myocardial 76
Poiseuille's law 63, 87, 171
Poisoning, carbon monoxide 66, 71
  drug overdosage 240
  renal damage in 202
Poliomyelitis 150
Polycythaemia 71, 88, 149, 182
Polyuria 216
Postrenal failure 201
Posture 136, 171
Potassium 25–8
  depletion 191–2
  intravenous dosage 35
  renal regulation of 26
  requirements 27
P-R interval 98
Prerenal failure 199
Pressure, arterial, age variation 78
  blood 76–9, 93
  blood, recording of 143
  central venous 79, 95
  continuous positive 164, 167
  cycling 113
  diastolic 76, 94
  generators, ventilator 109
  intrapleural 62, 80, 176
  intrathoracic 62, 75, 79
  filling, of ventricles 75
  left atrial 81, 84, 185
  mean 77
  partial, of gas 48
  perfusion 77
  pulmonary artery 80, 84
  pulmonary venous 80, 181
  pulmonary wedge 81, 84
  pulse 76
  receptors 84–5
  right atrium 84
  right ventricle 84
  systolic 76, 94
Propranolol 194, 239
Proteins, in diet 37
Pulmonary, artery banding 231
  atelectasis 129, 172
  blood flow 81

Index

Pulmonary—*cont.*
  blood volume 61
  collapse, active 173
  collapse, passive 174
  consolidation 129
  hypertension 182
  oedema 108, 130, 181
  vascular congestion 167, 182
  vascularity 130, 182
  vasculature 180–1
Purpura, Schönlein-Henoch 203
Pyelonephritis 204
Pyruvic acid 51, 57, 186

Q-T interval 101

Radiograph, in respiratory disease 130, 149
Radiographic technique 126
Ratio, inspiratory: expiratory 106
  respiratory exchange 65
  urine/plasma urea 208
  V_D/V_T 170
  ventilation: perfusion 65
Receptors, alpha-adrenergic 86
  beta-adrenergic 86
  chemo- 61, 85
  pressure 84
  stretch 85
Recordings, of fluid balance 138
Reflex, Moro 227
Relatives, nurse and 146
Renal, biopsy 207
  blood flow 199
  failure 58, 199, 206–212
  hypoplasia 204
  infarction 203
  parenchymal failure 201
  'shut down' 191, 197, 253
Reserpine 194
Resistance, airway 63, 171
  pulmonary vascular 81–2
  total peripheral 78, 89
  vascular 77, 78
  vessels 89

Resonium A 36
  calcium 211
Respiration, paradoxical 175, 223
Respiratory, centre 61, 150
  depressants 161
  disease 148
  distress syndrome 167
  exchange ratio 65
  failure 57, 72, 150, 245
  physiology in infants 68
  quotient 68
  stimulants 153, 241, 251
Respirometer 103, 107
Resuscitation, emergency 245
  trolley 146, 246, 254
Retrolental fibroplasia 69, 221
Ripple mattress 235

Salicylate, serum 242
Saline manometer 142
Sclerema 150, 221
Scleroderma 150
Schönlein-Henoch purpura 203
Septicaemia, epiglottitis 149
  gram-negative 17, 200
Septostomy, balloon 230
Servo-controlled incubator 144
Severinghaus electrode 53
Shock 200
  'irreversible' 193
  tissue perfusion in 90
Shunt, anatomical 170
  aorto-pulmonary 230
  capillary 170
  intra-pulmonary 65, 170
  left-to-right 182, 230
  right-to-left 182
  total 170
'Sick-cell' syndrome 23, 24
Siggaard-Andersen nomogram 54
Skin, care of 135, 162, 234
Sodium, bicarbonate dosage 57, 249
  low serum level 23
  'pump' 24
  re-absorption 200

Sodium—*cont.*
  renal regulation 23
  requirements 23
Solenoid valve 116, 123
Solutions, intravenous 34, 42
  priming for pump-oxygenator 185
Spasm, infundibular 194
Specific gravity, of urine 208
Sphincter, post-capillary 89
  pre-capillary 89
Sphygmomanometer 93, 143
Spironolactone 23
Sputum retention 152, 154
S–T segment 101
Standard bicarbonate 50, 225
Starling pump 123
Status epilepticus 150, 162, 237
Stenosis, aortic 180
Sterilization, of equipment 9, 19
Steroids, in laryngeal oedema 155, 166
  in shock 193
Stokes-Adams attack 247
Stridor 131, 149
  'congenital laryngeal' 151
Stroke volume 73
Subglottic stenosis 154
Surface tension 63, 219
Surfactant 62, 167, 219
Surgical emphysema 156–9, 177
Sympathetic nerves to heart 85–7
Syndrome, Guillain-Barré 150
  haemolytic-uraemic 203
  'low cardiac output' 193
  Mendelson 151, 165
  nephrotic 200
  Pierre-Robin 151, 152
  respiratory distress 167
  'sick cell' 24
  Waterhouse-Friderichsen 25
System, nervous 102

Tachycardia, cardiac output in 74, 99
  paroxysmal atrial 99, 192
  sinus 99
  ventricular 99, 192
Tamponade, cardiac 190
Temperature 104
  core 144, 172
  hypothalamus and 84
  measurement of 101, 104, 144
  recording 144, 224
Tetanus 238
Tetany, neonatal 29, 225
THAM 191
Thermometer 104, 144, 224
Thermistor 101, 103
Thermocouple 104, 144, 224
Thrombosis, intravascular 182, 197
Tidal volume 64, 107
Time constant, of lung 63
Tissue, exchange of fluid 89
  perfusion 101, 186
Tracheal, aspiration 141, 160
  dilators 141, 157
  intubation 153
  stricture 159
Tracheostomy 132, 140, 156–9
  decannulation 159
  incisions 157
  tubes 140, 158
Transducer 93, 95
Triggering, of ventilator 112
'Trocath' 177, 214
Tube feeding 137
Tube, intercostal 175
  nasotracheal 140
  orotracheal 140
  tracheostomy 140
Tubocurarine 161
Tubular necrosis 200
  ischaemic 201
  nephrotoxic 202

Ulceration of nasal septum 140, 155
Ultrasonic nebuliser 115, 220
Umbilical vein, catheterization of 137

Index

Unconscious patient 135–7, 162, 232–6
Unconsciousness, causes of 235
Underwater sealed drainage 139, 175
Uraemia 206
Urea, blood 200, 204, 206
  urine 207
  urine/plasma ratio 208
Uric acid 204
Urine, acid, in potassium depletion 26
  collection 136, 144, 210, 234
  concentration 200
  measurement of 33
  output 205, 210
  output, recording 136

Vagus nerve 85
Vein, brachial basilic 96
  cannulation of 137
  internal jugular 96
  subclavian 96
Venous, congestion 194
  return, during artificial ventilation 107
  return, factors affecting 79, 194
Ventilation, alveolar 64
  artificial 160–1
  artificial, physiology of 107
  assessment of 102
  control of 61
  in children 112
  mechanisms 62
  monitoring of 103, 106, 162
  perfusion ratio 65
  positive-positive 160, 167
  restriction of 195–6, 224
Ventilator, action of 108
  Amsterdam infant 116
  Barnet Mk. III 118
  Bird Mark 7 and 8 119
  Blease Pulmoflator Series 5000 122
  Bourns paediatric 123
  choice of 105
  cycling of 110, 112, 113
  Engström 123, 161
  expiratory phase 111
  inspiratory phase 108
  Loosco 116
  'lung' 105
  management of patient on 161
  monitoring of 162
  Starling pump 123
  sterilization 20
  tubing, support of 140
  weaning from 163
Viscosity, of blood 88
Vital capacity 64
Vitamin supplements 39
Volume, cycling 113
  end diastolic 74, 75
  end systolic 74, 75
  minute 162
  stroke 73
  tidal 64

Water, balance 210
  bath humidifier 116
  distribution in body 21
  in humidifiers 16
  intoxication 206, 218
  primary overload 24, 32
  requirements 22
Weaning, from ventilator 163
Weighing, bed 139, 210
  daily 139
Wheezing 148
Work, cardiac 76
Wright respirometer 103, 107

X-ray apparatus 126